Praise for
My Two Elaines and Marty Schreiber

Best Caregiver Books
Caring.com

100 Best Alzheimer's Books of All Time
BookAuthority

#2 Senior Social Media Influencers You Should Follow, 2018
Lively

Headliner Award, 2019
Milwaukee Press Club

Caregiver of the Week, August 2017
The Women's Alzheimer's Movement

Special Service Award, 2016
Alzheimer's Association

City of Milwaukee "Superhero," 2016
Milwaukee Press Club

"If you or someone you know is a caregiver, this is a must-read.
Your loved one really does become a different person. As I learned
from my mom's dementia, learning how to deal with her was key to
everyone's sanity. There are many helpful hints here."

—BONNIE BLAIR, five-time Olympic gold medalist

"At one moment this book is a heart-wrenching account of the devastating toll of Alzheimer's, and the next moment it is a heart-wrenching love story. The minute you are holding your breath at the brutality of the disease, Marty rescues you with a concrete, do-able message that can lead to lovely moments of joy. No health-care professional, family member, or caregiver should be without it."

—DAWN ADLER, director, Ovation Adult Day Services,
Milwaukee, Wisconsin, coauthor of *Illuminate:*
An Integrated Curriculum for Early
Memory Loss Programs

"Marty shares his personal story with dignity and grace. *My Two Elaines* helps the caregiver realize you must take care of yourself, have a sense of humor, and take advantage of help to survive the stressful days ahead. It is a great resource for families."

—LINDA CODY, director, Village Walk
Senior Living, Patchogue, New York

"Your book is now at the top of my list—written from the heart, rein-forcing yet honest."

—SUSAN M. GROSS, education and family care
specialist, Alzheimer's Association
North Central Texas Chapter

"This wonderful book gives a personal perspective of a couple's jour-ney with Alzheimer's disease as they reach out for help and support. The personal sharing, the compelling development of Marty, and his insights as a caregiver all provide for an important message."

—MICHAEL MALONE, MD, medical director, Aurora
Senior Services chair; Public Policy Committee,
American Geriatrics Society

"Marty has truly captured the essence of loving and caring for somebody with this disease. His book is insightful, thoughtful, heartwarming, and respectful. Marty's sense of humor and abundant patience surely are a blessing for Elaine."

—SCOTT MCFADDEN, president and CEO,
Lutheran Home and Harwood Place,
Milwaukee, Wisconsin

"To be complete, stories about Alzheimer's disease and caregiving must touch on both defeats and triumphs. In *My Two Elaines*, Governor Schreiber stirs the hearts of readers both with great suffering and great love inherent to the caregiving journey, lightening the load with humor. He introduces us not only to the woman he married and the person she became after Alzheimer's but also to the extraordinary individual who loves them both: her Marty."

—DANIEL C. POTTS, MD, FAAN, attending neurologist,
Tuscaloosa VA Medical Center, Alabama;
founder and president, Cognitive
Dynamics Foundation

"With poignant clarity and candor, Schreiber provides readers with insight into the often incomprehensible world of a person living with Alzheimer's disease as well as the many challenges faced by family caregivers. *My Two Elaines* is easily integrated into healthcare curriculum, sparking rich discussions related to dementia, caregiving, anticipatory grief, advance care planning, and community support services. Feedback has been overwhelmingly positive, with many learners expressing gratitude for the opportunity to gain a deeper understanding of the family caregiver experience."

—DR. STACY BARNES, director, Wisconsin
Geriatric Education Center,
Marquette University

"*My Two Elaines* demonstrates beautifully that the journey is not just for the person with the diagnosis but for the spouse and family as well, and that it is a journey to not attempt alone and unsupported. [Marty's] discussions will no doubt help those who may be afraid to admit they don't have it all under control. I highly recommend this book. It is a quick read that provides a lot of great advice that will decrease the learning curve immensely."

–TARA REED, author of *What to Do Between the Tears: A Practical Guide to Dealing with a Dementia or Alzheimer's Diagnosis in the Family*

"Marty Schreiber has written a book that is invaluable to the Alzheimer's community. His personal experience (and wisdom gained) as a caregiver is shared in such an honest and impactful way that it should be mandatory reading for all individuals who step forward in this capacity."

–DAVID SIMBRO, senior vice president, Northwestern Mutual; former member, Alzheimer's Association Board of Directors

"*My Two Elaines* provides real-life lessons about how to cope and survive each day with loving care, particularly when communication is lost. Marty helps caregivers work through their guilt and sheds light on making difficult decisions when professional care is needed for a loved one. Most of all, Marty brings us an amazing story of love, understanding, and hope. It is one of the most moving and powerful stories I've read."

–JULIE TOMBARI, administrator, New Day Adult Care Center, North Palm Beach, Florida

"I encourage my fellow health-care professionals to read and share this book."

"I only wish my father had this book to help him during my own mother's illness."

"This book is a narrative tool to help increase people's understanding of Alzheimer's disease and related dementias (ADRDs) and the caregiver experience. . . . There are few narratives from the male caregiving perspective, and this resource provides a unique opportunity to learn about their challenges. . . . In addition, the book can be used in training programs for direct care workers to increase knowledge and understanding levels on these topics."

MY TWO ELAINES

*Learning, Coping, and Surviving as an
Alzheimer's Caregiver*

~~~

MARTIN J. SCHREIBER

with CATHY BREITENBUCHER

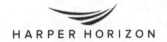

HARPER HORIZON

ISBN 978-0-7852-9170-1 (eBook)
ISBN 978-0-7852-9169-5 (HC)
ISBN 978-0-7852-9178-7 (SC)
ISBN 978-1-4041-2088-4 (CU)

Library of Congress Control Number: 2021951484

It wasn't until a few weeks ago that I really had to say, "Yes, I do have Alzheimer's." I had read of signs that indicate Alzheimer's, like getting overly upset for no reason and having trouble with names and directions. But I still didn't think it was a problem for me. But in hindsight ... for too long, I've been getting lost driving, having trouble keeping days straight and difficulties with names and schedules. Still, I still felt I could handle it—it won't get worse. But this morning, I started reading about the mid stage of Alzheimer's, in hopes of preparing myself better, and realized I'm not very far away. That is most scary! But I have to accept it.

—ELAINE'S LETTER TO HER "DEAR LOVED ONES,"
MARCH 11, 2009

Contents

Foreword

THE NAMES MARTIN AND Elaine Schreiber will ring a bell for many in Wisconsin, especially political watchers. The story they know is that of the state's thirty-ninth governor and his first lady. Since 1962 when Marty won his first political race for state senate, they were familiar faces on the political circuit, crisscrossing the state in campaigns for lieutenant governor, then for governor. They made an elegant couple, greeting Bobby Kennedy, President Carter, and other national leaders who came to Wisconsin. For almost thirty years, election night usually found the Schreibers side by side, watching the returns come in for one of Marty's races, accepting the victories and the defeats with grace. Later, when his own political career had finished, Marty became one of the state's best-known government-relations consultants.

This was the story I knew in the beginning, the one familiar to so many, but it is not the one you will find in the pages of this book. *My Two Elaines* is instead the story of what happened to the Schreibers later in life when Elaine began to show the first signs of Alzheimer's disease and then gradually, but surely, came under its grip.

Although this is the Schreibers' personal tale, many Americans will recognize the broad outlines. Alzheimer's disease is now the sixth leading cause of death in the United States, claiming more than 120,000 lives every year.[1] And the numbers are bound to rise as modern medicine helps us to live longer. Alzheimer's is one of the great health challenges facing mankind in the twenty-first century. It is also a disease that inspires a unique kind of dread. We find it terrifying to imagine a time when the body will continue to function but the mind will slip away.

So, in practical terms, *My Two Elaines* is an invaluable guide to millions who will face Alzheimer's in the role of patient or caregiver. In its pages, you will find a knowing and sympathetic guide to the day-to-day work of living with the disease. And it's important you have no illusions, for work it is.

Marty is clear about that.

When I first got to know the former governor in 2015 , I was struck by his honesty. Politicians are gregarious, but on their own terms. They spend so much of their time letting us see only the good qualities, the strong ones. On the campaign circuit, vulnerability may not count for much, but in everyday life, it is deeply underrated. It is the quality that infuses *My Two Elaines* with its power and makes it a valuable addition to the literature on Alzheimer's. To his great credit, Marty opens his life fully as a husband and Alzheimer's caregiver. He allows readers to see the sorrow, the frustration, and even the anger that comes from watching this disease destroy someone you love. He also describes the small moments of joy that even Alzheimer's cannot take away.

But it would not do justice to the book to file it away among the how-to or self-help guides. I read and enjoyed *My Two Elaines* most of all as a love story. The Schreibers' love for each other shines through on every page. It has endured the worst insults that Alzheimer's heaps on the living. It has endured even as the disease constructs a wall between the couple and the rich years they've shared.

In its raw honesty, this book itself is an act of love. Stories make us feel less alone in the world. Marty has generously given us his and Elaine's.

—Mark Johnson, Pulitzer Prize winner,
coauthor of *One in a Billion: The Story of Nic Volker
and the Dawn of Genomic Medicine*

Preface

I FELT COMPELLED TO write this book in the hope that relating my experience of caring for my wife, who was diagnosed with Alzheimer's disease in 2007, would help other caregivers learn, cope, and survive. That said, while sharing this message with other caregivers is my primary objective, those who looked over the manuscript told me they believed this book could help a wider audience as well. So, I invite husbands and wives, families and friends, to use it to better understand Alzheimer's, to learn how to assist caregivers, and to help patients experience moments of joy even as they daily face the overwhelming sadness of this disease.

Because I believe that maintaining a sense of humor is helping me bear up under the stress of Alzheimer's, at the beginning of several chapters, I've included some anecdotes that I hope make you laugh. If my icebreakers aren't your style, I beg your forgiveness as you focus on the book's central messages.

It wasn't until I was almost finished with the manuscript that I began finding many diaries, notes, and letters that Elaine had written at various times after her diagnosis. These writings sparked sadness as they led me to realize that at times, I hadn't been the best caregiver, yet they also brought joy to know that I'd made her feel happy and comforted too. Although we had prayed and cried together many times, until I read Elaine's own words, I never had a full comprehension of her emotions—her fears and anxieties, her love, and ultimately, her courage. It helped me understand how critically important I was to her as her lifeline as she faced her daunting future. I am so pleased I can share a fuller picture of Elaine by including her side of the story.

Many of the statistics cited in this book are from the Alzheimer's Association, which has led the world in Alzheimer's care, support, and research since 1980. For information and support, call the association's 24-7 helpline (1-800-272-3900) or visit https://www.alz.org.

Introduction

I MET MY FIRST Elaine in 1953, when we were both freshmen at
what is now called Milwaukee Lutheran High School in southeastern Wisconsin. My last name—Schreiber—and hers—
Thaney—put us pretty close in classroom seating.

My First Elaine helped me achieve each one of my successes
and stood by me in every one of my losses and illnesses. She
helped me pass biology at the University of Wisconsin-
Milwaukee. She worked as a secretary to put me through Marquette University Law School. She pushed our daughter, Kathy,
in a stroller while campaigning door-to-door for my first race in
1962; when I won, she won too. She celebrated with me later that
year when I was elected to the Wisconsin State Senate. Four
years later and pregnant, she kept four-year-old Kathy and our
son Marty, age three, neat and presentable during a station-
wagon tour of all seventy-two counties in Wisconsin in my race
for lieutenant governor. I lost and continued to serve in the state
senate.

I did win election as lieutenant governor in 1970, and eventually we had four children. In 1977, I became the thirty-ninth
governor of Wisconsin. There were more campaigns to run—for

governor in 1978 and 1982 and mayor of Milwaukee in 1988. I lost those, too, but I was experienced at not always coming out on top. As I've said many times in my life, my role in law school was to assure that there would be an upper 50 percent of the graduating class. Elaine uncomplainingly went to work as a teacher to get our family back on stable financial ground after my political run ended. I am profoundly grateful for her support.

We may have lost elections, but she never let me be defeated. In my second career, I've worked in insurance, publishing, and government affairs. The high of being a husband, a father, a grandfather, and now a great-grandfather surpasses any thrill I ever experienced in politics or business.

Elaine was as intelligent, kind, gracious, loving, understanding, self-sacrificing, and forgiving as any wife, mother, or grandmother could ever be. She cooked, kept house, raised the children, held dinner parties, dressed stylishly, took me to chemotherapy as I battled cancer, and sailed with me.

If it weren't for her, there wouldn't be me.

It was about 2005, when she was in her mid-sixties, that Elaine began to slip away from me. Her daily skills declined, and her interest in long-held hobbies withered. The time came when she couldn't drive without getting lost. Gradually, my constant helpmate became dependent on me for everything. Today, she does not cook, keep house, hold dinner parties, or dress herself. She got lost on our boat and in our home of twenty years, and eventually forgot her family, including me.

Even with Alzheimer's disease, Elaine remains as kind, gracious, loving, and self-sacrificing as any person could be. But she is not the same person. My First Elaine gave way to my Second Elaine.

I have hoped, laughed, and cried with both of them, just as anyone has with their spouse or loved one—and I now have had to acknowledge that the future will not unfold the way I thought it would.

My First Elaine and I shared love, hope, happiness, and dreams. As she became my Second Elaine, the dreams turned into nightmares because I was losing her. Happiness became hopelessness. Grieving and health issues (including depression and anxiety) replaced joy.

I greatly miss my First Elaine. My heart broke as she left me. It was so painful as this "new normal" enveloped us, with Alzheimer's destroying the memories we had created over decades. I still love her, of course, but in a quite different way. And I still want to make her happy, even when she is confused, unsettled, anxious, and much less aware of most things in life.

One day about five years into her disease, the Second Elaine asked me how we got together.

"Well," I told her, "when you were fourteen, I saw how pretty and smart and nice you were. I determined I wanted you for my wife, and if any other boys got within fifty feet of you, I bopped them on the head."

"You're a bullshitter," she said. My First Elaine would never have used language like that! When it came out, it was a bit shocking but funny, so I laughed, and she laughed. The new Elaine was speaking out. We shared an unexpected moment of joy.

"Well," I said, "let's just keep that between you and me."

"Oh no," she insisted. "It won't do any good. Everyone already knows."

IT IS SAID THAT there are more books written about Abraham Lincoln than any other subject in American nonfiction.[1] When your spouse has dementia, you might feel that our sixteenth president has given way to Dr. Alois Alzheimer, the German physician who was a pioneer in the study of memory loss. Before I became an Alzheimer's caregiver, I never imagined there was so much material out there—medical journals, memoirs, poetry, essays, and more. Sadly, with an estimated 6.2 million Americans aged sixty-five and older currently living with Alzheimer's and 13.8 million expected to be challenged by the disease by the year 2060, it's a growth industry.[2]

Over the course of my wife's eighteen-year struggle with Alzheimer's, I've looked at plenty of those books. I didn't benefit much from the bookish science stuff or the bullet-point how-tos. Not one of the books I read conveyed the ugly truth about caregiving: that it can destroy you—even kill you—if you go about it wrong. I hope this book speaks to you so that you can help your partner on his or her Alzheimer's journey, be the best caregiver possible, and survive.

What I have learned over the past almost-two decades will, I hope, make a difference in your life and that of your loved one. I have hiked up the Alzheimer's mountain, have identified its dangerous areas, and am meeting you now on the way back down as you begin your own climb. Please, don't take another step until you hear what I have to say.

As you know—unfortunately, tragically—you are at a moment when it is impossible for you to avoid taking this journey. You are unable to turn back. Your health, your spirit, your very life all are in danger unless you learn more about what lies ahead. By knowing where the hazards are, you can avoid some of the mistakes I have made and, in doing so, better help your spouse deal with this disease.

In the United States, more than one in nine people aged sixty-five and older have Alzheimer's. Statistically speaking, it is a woman's disease—almost two-thirds of Americans with Alzheimer's are female. That's 3.8 million individual tragedies as of

2021.[3] Yet, when you find out that your partner has Alzheimer's, you feel utterly alone. You used to share your problems with and get support from this person, but now you can't. Your partner is no longer your partner; he or she is your responsibility. Suddenly, you don't know where to turn. So, you dig in your heels, convinced that you can outlast this disease. Especially if you're the man of the household, you may feel you have a tough-guy image to maintain. You worked hard, raised a family, built a business or two—or maybe even governed a state.

For men who are caregivers to wives with Alzheimer's, the definition of manhood changes. It's not about being tough; it's about being smart. It's going to be hard for you to change your thinking, I know. The real way to demonstrate your manhood—and I learned this the hard way—is to not try to go it alone. Asking for help doesn't mean you're less of a man.

This advice applies to female caregivers as well. Often, wives are used to doing it all—juggling the family's schedules, keeping the house in order, doing the bulk of shopping and meal preparation, and working outside the home too. Taking care of someone with dementia makes a sizable dent in the time and energy available for those other necessary tasks. Asking for help doesn't mean you're less of a wife.

Let me be your trail guide. I will tell you why it's essential to reach out for help. Many of these thoughts will be found throughout the book in notes titled "What I wish I'd known." I'll also show you how to cope in notes labeled "What I wish I'd done."

Along the way, I'll try to teach you how allowing yourself moments of joy can help you survive. And I'll do it with a little humor. Without humor, you'll go nuts.

On your journey, your beloved partner will be replaced by someone with the same name in the same body. Your loved one's mind will be even more different than you can imagine. As time passes, his or her memory will be erased to such a degree that most of the memories of your life together are partially missing or completely gone. You will experience someone behaving and talking in a manner different from the person you have known and loved. Can there be anything more painful? Probably not. I call it death by a thousand cuts. But know this: there are Band-Aids for these cuts—resources and help of which you must take advantage.

As a caregiver, you will do heroic work. You may be thinking, *Me? A hero?* I say, "Yes! A hero!" Even though your efforts won't be enough to stop the disease from stealing your partner, the deeds you will perform as you continue to care for and love your partner are heroic.

No job or responsibility you've ever shouldered will be as challenging as this new role. When your partner has Alzheimer's, almost without thinking, you put his or her needs above yours. Eventually you realize you've gone from 100 percent spouse to 100 percent caregiver. Your skills and patience will be tested to the point where you think you, too, are losing your mind. Being a caregiver to someone who no longer knows your name is the last thing any of us think of when we vow "in sickness and in health." But here you are. It hurts, and it takes its toll, more so when you don't get help.

Seldom does anyone become a hero without preparation. Not the soldiers in the D-Day invasion force, not the astronauts in the *Apollo 13* crew, not even the local high school quarterback. Starting right now, you must step aside from all the busyness of life to understand yourself as a caregiver-hero. The sooner you focus on your new role truthfully, the better you can cope. You owe it to yourself and to your loved one to get this right. In the end, all you can say is that you did your best. That makes you a hero.

My heart goes out to you. But remember: learn about Alzheimer's, learn how to cope with it, learn how to survive.

MY TWO
ELAINES

My Marty, who is and always has been my strength and comfort. I thank God every day for his understanding, loving ways, patience, good humor, hard work. He has made possible not only four wonderful children and a wonderfully exciting and busy life for me, but also helped so many others throughout his lifetime. He has a true gift for making those around him feel good about themselves, laugh at his jokes, and grow into stronger people. I thank you for that, hon, as I've benefited the most.

—Elaine's letter to her "dear loved ones,"
March 11, 2009

꧁꧂

CHAPTER 1

When Marty Met Elaine

I F YOU BELIEVE IN love at first sight, then I fell in love with
Elaine Ruth Thaney in the fall of 1953. We were freshmen in
Latin class at Lutheran High School, which was located at Thir-
teenth and Vine Streets, just west of where Interstate 43 now
makes its way from downtown to the North Shore suburbs. In
those postwar years, enrollment was growing so quickly that the
school building, constructed in 1908, was bursting at the seams.
Old army barracks were added to the property to provide enough
classroom space. It didn't matter that there were hundreds of
girls at Lutheran; I knew right away Elaine was the one for me.
Apparently she thought so, too, because neither of us dated anyone else throughout high school.

At the start of our junior year, our school, which had split off
from the original institution and was now called Milwaukee Lutheran High School, moved to a newly constructed building in a
sparsely populated area on the northwest side of Milwaukee.
That same year, Disneyland opened in California, Jonas Salk's
polio vaccine was declared safe and effective, and in Montgom-
ery, Alabama, Rosa Parks refused to give up her seat on a bus to

a white passenger. Change was everywhere, except when it came to Elaine and me. We were in love.

I was raised on Center Street near North Twenty-Fifth Street, in a small house behind my father's real estate office. He had served a term in the Wisconsin State Assembly and later was elected to the Milwaukee Common Council. Our house featured just one bedroom, so my father, who was well trained as a carpenter, put partitions in the attic to create bedrooms for me, my older sister, and my kid brother.

Elaine grew up on Grant Boulevard in the Sherman Park area, which is still a desirable neighborhood in Milwaukee because of its beautiful brick and quarry-stone homes. The first time I drove her there, I saw these magnificent residences, and I couldn't believe how big they were. *Wow*, I thought to myself. Then she said, "My house is on the other side of the street," and it was a very modest structure. There went any delusions I might have had about marrying for money! Her father owned a company that made concrete blocks. He worked hard to keep the business going so he could support his family. He would tell Elaine, "God made me rich with five children."

Elaine was the oldest child. A bright girl, she was one of those kids you loved to hate because it seemed she always got As and never needed to study. But she had well-rounded interests—she was selected as a cheerleader, was a member of the synchronized swimming team, and even took up the drums. She later told me she did that so she could be with me in the school band; it didn't hurt that a set of drumsticks cost maybe seventy-five cents, well within her family's budget. I played second chair clarinet.

It was rare that I outshone Elaine. When I was elected as a class officer, it was largely because she helped by painting clever red-and-blue campaign signs that looked like wanted posters.

Elaine's generous spirit was evident throughout her teenage years. When I turned sixteen, she took up a collection from our friends to rent a park pavilion for a surprise birthday party. From the money our classmates chipped in, she proudly presented me with water skis that cost eighteen dollars—quite a sum in the mid-1950s. When she turned sixteen a few months later, she got her first real job, at a dry-cleaning business managed by an elderly woman. Knowing that this lady had no relatives, one year Elaine insisted that we buy a small Christmas tree and take it to her.

After high school, Elaine headed to what was then called Concordia Teachers' College (now Concordia University Chicago), a Lutheran school in River Forest, Illinois. I wanted to be either an attorney or a minister, and I went to a different Lutheran school, Valparaiso University, in northwestern Indiana. By car, our colleges were about an hour and a half apart. Long-distance phone calls cost something like $1.75 for three minutes, which was never long enough for me. I was worried I might lose her to a boy at Concordia.

With money tight in her family, Elaine transferred after her freshman year to a public school, the University of Wisconsin's main campus in Madison. I had given up any aspirations I had to become a minister, so I left Valparaiso University to enroll at the University of Wisconsin–Milwaukee. We were back in the same state again, but still an hour and a half apart. After a year in Madison, Elaine decided to join me at UW-Milwaukee. That was my saving grace, personally and academically. Without Elaine sitting next to me in botany and biology, I never could have passed those classes. She had a keen mind in the classroom.

But Elaine put her education on hold for me. After our junior year of college, I was accepted across town at Marquette University, into a program that gave me a jump start on law school. Elaine took a full-time job as a secretary (and I worked construction over the summers) to save money so we could get married, which we did on June 3, 1961. I had two years of law school remaining.

They say timing is everything, and I lucked out in the spring of 1962. My parents had recently cosigned the mortgage for a $7,500 duplex on West Monroe Street near Twenty-Fifth and Center. Then a vacancy occurred in the state senate, in the district where we lived, giving me the opportunity to run for office. One of my opponents in the four-man primary was Fred Kessler, who, believe it or not, had been a classmate of ours at Milwaukee Lutheran. He had been elected to the state assembly in 1960 at the age of twenty.

My dad was serving as a Milwaukee alderman, so I benefited from his name recognition with the voters. But my real advantage in the primary was Elaine. She took it upon herself to go downtown to the election commission office for the names of newly registered voters, of which there were hundreds. Then, she used maps and lists of polling places to write postcards to tell each new voter exactly where to vote. I have fond memories of Elaine's enthusiasm as she sat on our living room floor, surrounded by piles of postcards that needed to be hand-addressed and personalized. I considered it rather risky because—let's face it—mistakes could be made or a person might just vote for the other candidate! She proved to be an astute campaign worker as I squeaked past Fred by 350 votes—a victory at age twenty-three that charted our whole life. Two months later in the general election, I received 76 percent of the vote.

No time to celebrate, though. I was still wrapping up law school. After I took my oath of office in January 1963, I attended the Tuesday through Thursday legislative sessions, which meant two nights a week in Madison. Elaine had her hands full with our young daughter, Kathy, and we were expecting again—

our son Marty was born in April 1963. In 1964, I faced only token opposition in the general election.

Our third child was on the way in 1966 when I was running for lieutenant governor. The job paid $7,500 a year, compared to the $8,900 salary of a state senator. Elaine didn't bat an eye over that potential pay cut; she knew my goal was to become governor. It was obvious she was willing to do anything for me, including encouraging me to plan campaign events for late September, despite the conflict with our baby's due date. I had early-morning campaign appearances scheduled for September 28 in Beloit, about an hour southwest of Milwaukee, with plans to be home by early afternoon. Before I left home at 4:30 a.m., I asked Elaine if she was okay.

"I'm fine," she said. "You go."

Around 10:00 a.m., our daughter Kristine was ready to enter our hectic world. Elaine walked herself to the nearby St. Joseph Hospital—where she herself had been born in 1939—and soon I got a call at the library where I was speaking, to tell me that our baby daughter had arrived.

I lost that election and went back to the state senate, retaining my seat in the 1968 election and biding my time for another shot at lieutenant governor in 1970. By then, the state constitution had been changed so that the candidates for lieutenant governor and governor ran together. So, running in 1970 with Patrick Lucey at the top of the ticket, we were elected. One newspaper article described me as the Lucey ticket putting its best foot forward. Elaine was so proud and excited for me. She made our daughters' dresses and her own for the inauguration. In 1974, the Lucey-Schreiber team won reelection. Our family celebrated again in 1975, when our son Matt was born.

In case you don't remember the 1976 presidential election, Jimmy Carter narrowly defeated the Republican incumbent,

Gerald R. Ford. That meant Carter could, among other things, pick a new ambassador to Mexico. Carter nominated his fellow Democrat, Patrick Lucey, and after the United States Senate confirmed Lucey, I succeeded him as governor on July 6, 1977. We held an open house at the Wisconsin Executive Residence the next day–7/7/77–and, despite a hot summer sun, the line stretched down the driveway and out into the street. We shook thousands of hands!

The 1970s were a roller coaster of a decade for us, with my campaigning all over the state and my duties in Madison. At one point, we had a teenager, a baby, and two kids in between. How Elaine held it all together and made it look so effortless is beyond me. Did I mention that she also went back to college and completed her education degree in 1974?

As a kid, I had prayed that I'd someday be governor. Maybe I should have prayed for five four-year terms–I mean, why not go for it?–because my time in office proved to be much shorter than I had hoped. In the 1978 election, a political newcomer named Lee S. Dreyfus ran an unconventional campaign and beat me with about 55 percent of the vote. My, could he orate! I moved on to an executive position at Sentry Insurance in Stevens Point in central Wisconsin, and we bought a forty-four-acre hobby farm in the next county over. Our daughter Kathy stayed in Madison to finish high school, but our three younger children moved with us and enjoyed the slower pace of country living. We had animals galore. When our goat gave birth to triplet kids (a somewhat rare event), we named them Breakfast, Lunch, and Dinner. Meanwhile, Elaine and her friend Barbara opened an antiques and crafts store in the farm's restored granary building. Although it barely broke even, she enjoyed it.

Elaine was upbeat and positive in every campaign. She always told me, "Don't be afraid of losing." I guess that was good advice

because I didn't make it out of the primary in the 1982 guberna-
torial election. A couple of years later, we headed home to Milwaukee, where I hoped to be elected mayor in 1988, but I fell
short in the general election. The major rap against me, as I recall, was that I was too nice to be mayor.

Over the next few years, we worked hard to relaunch our
careers—Elaine as a teacher and me as a public-affairs consultant.
Elaine even went back to college and earned a master's of education when she was fifty-six years old. She gave her heart to the
at-risk preschoolers at the Silver Spring Neighborhood Center
on Milwaukee's northwest side and later led a successful capital
campaign to benefit that organization. Because of Elaine's devotion, Silver Spring named its childhood development center for
her, an honor that was read into the Congressional Record by
United States Representative Gwendolynne Moore.

All the while, the kids grew up and moved out. Having married so young, we were empty nesters by our early fifties. We
found fulfillment as volunteers and board members for organizations around town. Such good times!

We thought they would last forever.

PART 1

Learning About Alzheimer's Disease

I'm so lucky he is a good cook and seems to enjoy making healthy and delicious meals. It's a good thing as my Alzheimer's isn't getting any better, so cooking and baking with steps that need to work are no longer easy for me. I hate to think I am getting worse, but I must be.

—ELAINE'S FLORIDA JOURNAL,
MARCH 31, 2012

CHAPTER 2

❦

Diagnosis

M Y FIRST EXPERIENCE WITH Alzheimer's was in 1978, when I was campaigning for governor. One bright fall day, I was giving a speech in Eau Claire, a college town in northwestern Wisconsin. It was essentially the same stump speech I'd been using all over the state to warm applause. Afterward, I was shaking some hands when an elderly gentleman came up to me. "That was the worst god-awful speech I ever heard," he snarled.

His wife followed behind quickly, wearing an embarrassed look. She apologized several times. "Governor, you've got to understand," she pleaded. "He's old and senile, and all he ever does is repeat whatever he hears everyone else say."

WHEN YOU LEARN THAT your loved one has Alzheimer's disease, it's the beginning of the end. It's easy to say that the diagnosis marks both an end and a beginning, and to a degree that's true. There's a "before" and an "after" to this news. But one part of your life doesn't instantly come to an end while another part magically crops up to take its place.

17

Dementia is a general term for a decline in mental ability severe enough to interfere with daily life. Not every kind of dementia is Alzheimer's; however, some forms of dementia, such as dementia with Lewy bodies and Creutzfeldt-Jakob disease, are equally devastating and fatal. Some people have what's called mixed dementia, which most commonly refers to the combination of Alzheimer's and another type of dementia.

On the other hand, people can have temporary symptoms of dementia after a stroke or because of medical conditions, including depression, urinary tract infections, thyroid problems, vitamin deficiencies, or adverse drug reactions. Issues such as these often can be successfully treated. So if a loved one is confused and anxious, don't panic and think the worst. *Have a doctor check for all possible explanations.*

Alzheimer's is the best-known, most common form of dementia. It accounts for 60 percent to 80 percent of all dementia cases.[1] It is unrelenting and irreversible, and it can drag on for years before it kills someone you love dearly. There. I just said what we all fear the most. This time around, I'm not being a BSer.

For those with dementia, the most fearful time may be that period when they know they're losing their minds and worry what the future outcome will be. It's a horrible thing to witness. One of the worst of these episodes in Elaine's and my journey was when she was preparing one of her favorite German meals for several friends who had come to our home for dinner. Although she'd been using these recipes for years, she got all mixed up and left out some of the ingredients. The food was inedible. But far worse was the desperate and sad look on Elaine's face as she understood why this was happening.

When something like that occurs, instinctively you help your partner more, or you start ordering pizza every night. Instead of addressing what's really going on, you just adapt. You sort of get used to it—and that's a form of denial. Months pass, and maybe you mention it to the doctor.

By the time you go to an Alzheimer's specialist, you have a pretty good sense of what's happening with your partner. Why else would you have made that appointment?

A diagnosis of Alzheimer's presents a real ethical challenge for doctors and caregivers. Is it better for the patient to know or to not know? It's a topic of such importance that the Alzheimer's Association issued a ten-page Special Report in its 2015 *Alzheimer's Disease Facts and Figures* resource. A study cited in the report found that only 45 percent of people with Alzheimer's were ever told of the diagnosis. Experts say there are benefits to knowing. These include having the time to make financial plans and the opportunity to be educated about and have access to support services.[2]

For us, the news wasn't a big shock based on the symptoms Elaine had been showing. As far back as 2005, when Elaine was sixty-five years old, she told a psychiatrist that she'd had concerns about her memory for a couple of years already. She explained that she sometimes had difficulty driving; when she got confused, she needed to stop the car to regain her sense of direction. Cognitive tests revealed a mixed bag; some memory skills were ranked as "average" and some "low average." None of those scores were in the "impaired" range.

In 2007, the doctor began to dig deeper. For one thing, he ordered an MRI of the brain. The scan didn't particularly point to trouble; in fact, it ruled out the possibility that Elaine had had a stroke. But her behavior was telling us that her brain was changing. Doctor appointments became more frequent.

At one appointment, she mentioned that she was having trouble remembering what she'd read, whether it was in newspapers or novels. She had all but given up on reading. At another appointment, she was able to easily give the receptionist her date of birth, but five minutes later in the exam room, she couldn't come up with it at all. At that point, she was given a different cognitive test called the Mini-Mental State Exam (MMSE). It was similar to the assessment she'd been given before: repeat a short list of words, name the current month, copy a drawing—that kind of thing. The scoring tops out at thirty, and while health-care professionals disagree on where the cutoffs should be,[3] we were told that people in the thirty to twenty-eight range were considered to have normal cognitive ability, those in the twenty-seven to twenty-five range had possible mild cognitive impairment, and so on down the line. Elaine scored a twenty-eight.

People with Alzheimer's can and do function well in the early stages of the disease. Just because you were diagnosed on Tuesday doesn't mean you can't put together a perfectly good sandwich or spreadsheet on Thursday. A year or two from Thursday? That's another matter.

As for Elaine, at the time of her diagnosis, she still took care of her basic needs, managed the house, and was socially engaged. On the surface, she was still the gracious first lady of Wisconsin who had welcomed artists, championship sports teams, Lillian Carter, and even the Crown Princess of Norway to the Wisconsin Executive Residence. If you didn't ask how long she'd stay at a twenty-eight or how she'd behave at a twenty-two, you could be lulled into thinking, *This isn't so bad.*

What I Wish I'd Known

A person with Alzheimer's will experience diminished mental capabilities at a rate of two to four points per year on the MMSE scale.[4] But it doesn't happen in a predictable way.

Still, the diagnosis was a milestone event: it came with her first prescription for an Alzheimer's drug, Aricept (donepezil). It's an oral medication that works to temporarily alter the brain's chemistry so that nerve cells can continue to trade information with one another. The doctor also recommended that she have a neurological evaluation.

Later that year, soon after Elaine turned sixty-eight, I sought out the best neurologist I could find at the Medical College of Wisconsin in Milwaukee. The examination and tests only confirmed what we had been told before:

Alzheimer's.

Beyond that, I honestly don't remember what words the doctor used. I'm sure he didn't say, "There is no hope" or "This is fatal." I already knew the one absolute about Alzheimer's: no one survives it. I do recall him emphasizing the importance of socialization, Aricept, and another drug called Namenda (memantine) to temporarily improve symptoms, plus daily exercise and a glass of red wine every night. Jokingly, I said that Elaine was two weeks behind on the exercise and two months ahead on the red wine.

We didn't need a third opinion. I respected the doctors we had. We left the clinic clinging to the notion that we could set our own course and somehow slow down the Alzheimer's death march. Like the good teacher she was (and in spite of her current difficulties with reading), Elaine headed to the library for every Alzheimer's book she could get her hands on. She devoured them, taking note after note almost as if she could beat the disease based on the number of books she read and notes she made. It also seemed that she was doing some type of penance or seeking forgiveness for the problems she knew she would later cause.

Deep down, she knew how bad it was going to get. She was dealing with the painful realization that she was going to lose her memory, her independence, her dignity, and eventually her life. Out loud, she worried that she would be abandoned. Would I still love her? Would I still take care of her?

"When I get to be a burden," she'd say, "you can put me away." Many nights, we cried ourselves to sleep.

SCIENTISTS HAVE BEEN STUDYING memory loss for better than a hundred years. In 1906, Alois Alzheimer first lectured on "an unusual disease of the cerebral cortex" that he had observed.[5] Ever since—particularly since 1980, when the Alzheimer's Association was founded—some of the brightest minds in medicine have worked to unravel this terrible disease.

Tremendous progress has been made over the past generation in treating many other diseases. Childhood cancer is a great example. The American Cancer Society says the overall five-year survival rate has climbed from about 58 percent in the mid-1970s to more than 80 percent today.[6]

But when it comes to Alzheimer's, we're hardly better off today than we were a hundred years ago. Most babies who were born in Alois Alzheimer's time didn't live past the age of fifty, according to the National Institute on Aging.[7] Meanwhile, babies born in the United States today are projected to live to just under seventy-nine years of age, according to the Centers for Disease Control and Prevention.[8] That longer lifespan gives Alzheimer's more of an opportunity to develop. And then there are the baby boomers, reaching age sixty-five at the rate of about ten thousand a day—a figure estimated to continue until the year 2030.[9] So the race is on to find a cure.

It takes years for any drug—such as those that blessedly have improved childhood cancer survival—to be approved for use in the United States by the Food and Drug Administration (FDA).

Contrary to what you might think, the FDA itself does not develop drugs. That happens in universities, hospitals, and pharmaceutical labs all over the world. For those of us without a scientific mind, the process seems ridiculously tedious: develop a theory, design a way to test it, run into a dead end, reexamine the theory, design a new test, run into a dead end, and on and on until you hit on something.

Once lab studies produce promising data, drug developers have to submit what's called an Investigational New Drug (IND) application to the FDA's Center for Drug Evaluation and Research (CDER). According to the FDA's website, CDER's mission is to "ensure that drugs marketed in this country are safe and effective. CDER doesn't test drugs, although the Center's Office of Testing and Research does conduct limited research in the areas of drug quality, safety, and effectiveness."[10] And I thought state government was a bureaucracy!

Only after an IND application is approved can the drug's sponsor begin testing on humans. Clinical trials are funded by pharmaceutical companies and medical device manufacturers, academic medical centers, foundations or individuals, organizations such as the Alzheimer's Association, or governmental agencies.

According to the National Institutes of Health, there are four phases to a clinical trial:

1. "Researchers test the drug or treatment in a small group of people" for the first time to evaluate its safety, determine a safe dosage range, and identify side effects.
2. "The new drug or treatment is given to a larger group of people" to see if it is effective and to further evaluate its safety.
3. "The new drug or treatment is given to large groups of people . . . to confirm its effectiveness, monitor side

effects, compare it with standard or similar treatments, and collect information that will allow the new drug or treatment to be used safely."

4. After the drug or treatment has been approved, "researchers track its safety in the general population" and gather more information on the drug's effect and optimal use.[11]

Sometimes a drug doesn't even make it through all the phases of a clinical trial. End of story. Back to the drawing board.

From 2002 to 2012, a total of 244 Alzheimer's drugs were tested with exactly one successfully completing the trials process and being approved by the FDA.[12] One!

So far, the drugs that have been approved by the FDA for use in treating Alzheimer's only slow the worsening of symptoms of the disease. They're effective for about six to twelve months, on average, for about half of the individuals who take them. Unfortunately, they don't treat the underlying disease or delay its progression. And only five such drugs are in use. That includes one that got the okay in 2014, which was a combination of two previously approved drugs.[13] Before that, the last time an Alzheimer's drug was approved for use in the United States was 2003.[14]

There you have it: the cold, hard truth that despite the gallant efforts of scientists around the world, there currently is no cure or even a decent way to slow down the brain-damaging effects of Alzheimer's. When your partner is diagnosed, you don't do yourself any favors by sticking your head in the sand. I hate to tell you, but it's going to get worse. It just is.

Alzheimer's doesn't stand still. Your partner will become someone you don't know. And you will become someone you don't recognize: a caregiver. At first, you don't call yourself that. You're simply a spouse who is caring for a loved one who is confused. But then without realizing it, and with no ability to stop this transformation, you morph from being a full-time partner into a full-time caregiver.

What I Wish I'd Done

Right away, I should have taken full advantage of all that the Alzheimer's Association has to offer. Besides support groups, there is individual counseling, plus online tools and information.

Sometimes, a person's decline is the steady, annoying but nonemergency drip-drip-drip of the bathroom faucet at 3:00 a.m. At other times, it's as if you're filling the watering can for the garden, you turn your back for a moment, and when you look again, the water is overflowing the can and creating a muddy mess. Big declines can sometimes occur if there are additional medical issues, such as a urinary tract infection.

We're a nation of doers. We aim high, and we despise failure. We keep score on the sports field and in the political arena. We look at a problem—such as that drippy bathroom faucet—and we figure it out. Alzheimer's can't be fixed, not yet anyway. But take heart: help is available so you can meet the challenge of life as a caregiver.

About three years after Elaine's diagnosis, one of the nurses at the neurologist's office asked me whether I'd joined any support groups. Who, me? I'm from that generation of men who weren't supposed to even have feelings, much less show them in public. Does the name Edmund Muskie ring a bell? He was a fine US senator from Maine, a leading candidate for the Democratic presidential nomination in 1972. But his bid fell apart on a snowy

New Hampshire morning when he denounced a publication that, among other slander, was critical of his wife. Some reports asserted that Muskie cried as he defended his wife, while Muskie himself claimed the falling snowflakes were responsible for the moisture on his face. Either way, opponents used the incident to claim Muskie was too emotional to run the country. He withdrew from the race not long after.[15]

As for me, I wasn't man enough to know I needed help to deal with my wife's health problem. My feeling was I didn't need a pity party. The problem with that attitude was that I didn't know what Alzheimer's support groups were all about. I wrongly thought I'd be sitting in a circle of weepy people trying to one-up one another's stories about their loved ones' behaviors.

I was doing fine (I thought). I'd be okay (I thought). But as we've all learned from Proverbs 16:18, pride goeth before the fall.

I'd be so lost without you—so please continue to take good care of yourself for me as well as for you.

—A NOTE FROM ELAINE
TO MARTY, 2013

CHAPTER 3

Danger on the Trail: How Alzheimer's Can Harm Your Health

E VER HEAR THE ONE about the hippopotamus and the butterfly who fell in love? As the hippo begins thinking about proposing and consummating the marriage, he quickly realizes he has a problem. So, he seeks out the wise old owl for advice.

The owl says, "I can see that this is troubling you. You've come to the wisest animal for advice. Here's your answer: what you've got to do is turn yourself into a butterfly."

The hippo starts to walk away but quickly realizes that he doesn't know just how he can do that. He returns to Mr. Owl and says, "I would do anything for my dear loved one. Please tell me, how can I change myself into a butterfly?"

"Sorry, buster," the owl replies. "I just determine policy."

LIKE THAT OWL, NO matter how wise you think you are, Alzheimer's has truths about it that you cannot change. Your spouse is going to get worse, mentally and physically. No one's got the answer to that. And you're likely to suffer mental and physical harm too. That shouldn't come as a big shocker because caregiving is a continuous process that puts unprecedented demands on your time, energy, and emotions. You cannot afford to be as arrogant as that owl.

If it makes you feel any better, you are not alone. It is estimated that in 2018, there were 16.2 million Americans providing unpaid care for people with Alzheimer's and other forms of dementia.[1] If you think 16.2 million sounds like a lot of people, you're right. It's ten-and-a-half times the US workforce of Walmart![2]

All those tasks you take on—out of love, concern, and a sense of responsibility—add up to an average of almost twenty-two hours per week. So nationwide, caregivers provided 18.5 billion hours of unpaid assistance in 2018. That's billion with a *b*.[3]

Here's another way of looking at what caregivers do: The federal minimum wage is $7.25 an hour. According to the Alzheimer's Association, data from the US Department of Labor reports home health aides' salaries averaged $18.02 an hour in 2018. The care you're providing must be worth more than what a fast-food worker makes, right? But maybe it's not as valuable as that of a trained professional health aide. So average those two salaries, and your work is worth $12.64 an hour. Of course, you're not in it for the money. But if all of us caregivers banded together, we'd have provided roughly $233.9 billion worth of care in 2018.[4]

Caregiving for people with dementia cuts across every demographic group you can think of. It is the job of the well-educated (approximately 40 percent have at least a college degree) as well as those with modest incomes (41 percent have a household income of fifty thousand dollars or less).[5]

One-third of Alzheimer's caregivers are, like me, over the age of sixty-five.[6] But some caregivers are young children. A 2005 study by the National Alliance for Caregiving found that approximately 250,000 kids in this country between the ages of eight and eighteen provide help to persons with Alzheimer's or another form of dementia.[7]

As you become an unpaid Alzheimer's caregiver, you do so without the benefit of training. Those professional home health aides I mentioned a minute ago? Federal regulations require seventy-five hours of training to get a job with a Medicare-certified home health agency, according to the Paraprofessional Healthcare Institute. (In my home state of Wisconsin, it's 120 hours).[8] For family caregivers, though, it's learning on the job, a baptism by fire.

Being an Alzheimer's caregiver takes a tremendous toll, but it happens in such a gradual way that you may not notice how harmful it is to you. Exercise? Eat healthy? Who has time for that? Managing your own health can be that "one more thing" you can't squeeze into a day that's already filled up with doctor appointments, newly inherited household chores, and possibly your own job responsibilities.

Trudging up the Alzheimer's mountain can sap all your physical and emotional strength. But I am here to tell you that you must make it a priority to be healthy yourself in order to be an effective caregiver. This is not negotiable. How do you keep yourself healthy? You get help. You take classes. You talk to people who have been through this. You cannot do it alone, as I tried to do. The proof is in the numbers and illustrated by my own experience.

Consider this: people with Alzheimer's who are sixty-five and older survive, on average, four to eight years after their diagnosis. Some live with the disease as long as twenty years.[9] When you give up a healthy lifestyle as a result of your caregiving burden, you're stacking the odds against yourself, leaving you with the sickening possibility that your partner with Alzheimer's will outlive you. That's got to be one of the cruelest twists of this terrible disease.

Maybe you've read the "Twelve Steps for Caregivers" by Carol J. Farran and Eleanora Keane-Hagerty, who have studied and written about Alzheimer's and caregiving for years. It's based on the many twelve-step programs for people with addictions and has been around since 1989, when it was published in an Alzheimer's-related medical journal, and it still pops up on websites, blogs, and social media. Right there in black and white it says a caregiver should recognize this: "I need to take care of myself."[10] It was good advice twenty-five years ago, and it's good advice today.

Think of the emergency instructions you get on an airplane—you have to put on your own oxygen mask before you can help others with theirs. No matter how much you love your partner, you can't take good care of him or her if you don't first take good care of yourself. I didn't realize how important that was until it was almost too late. I don't want that to happen to you.

What I Wish I'd Known

Chronic stress experienced by Alzheimer's caregivers may shorten their lives by as much as four to eight years.

When Elaine was well, and even after she first was diagnosed, I'd work out many weekday mornings with my friends. But as her mental decline continued, her body clock was affected, and that threw off my own sleep. If she was awake, I felt I, too, should be awake to make sure she wasn't wandering around or doing something unsafe. Sometimes, she'd ask and reask me questions, and they were not any old questions. Instead, her queries packed an emotional punch. "Are we married?" "Do we have children?" "Do I have Alzheimer's?" "Is it bad?" "Why do I have it?" Just try getting back to sleep after that!

By the time we got up for the day, many times she'd be confused and agitated, and I'd be exhausted and cranky. I simply couldn't leave her home alone in the morning while I went to the health club. One missed workout led to another and another and, well, the theme from *Rocky*, the *William Tell* Overture, and "On, Wisconsin!" combined wouldn't have provided enough inspiration to push me out the door. Over the span of a year and a half, I gained twenty pounds.

Elaine, meanwhile, also put on weight, probably eight or ten pounds. Sometimes, she couldn't remember whether she'd eaten lunch. When in doubt, she'd make herself a peanut butter and jelly sandwich.

Carrying that extra weight—and I don't just mean the pounds—meant I couldn't even walk up the stairs at home or my office without having to stop and catch my breath. Even when I was merely walking, I often got short of breath. (My temper ran short too. More on that in chapter 5.)

I already was a cancer survivor, having been diagnosed in 2006 with non-Hodgkin's lymphoma. I went through six cycles of chemotherapy over a six-month period with side effects that included low energy, nausea, and hair loss. Even so, I remained confident that the treatment would work. And it did. So while I hated the idea of more clinics and exams for myself, I had to get some answers. The doctors quickly focused on a variety of heart issues.

Over a three-and-a-half-year span, from 2009 through late 2012, I underwent several procedures and also had a pacemaker installed. Still, I never felt quite right. I rang up more than $260,000 in medical bills as various doctors took their turns examining me, ordering tests and lab work, and even having me admitted. My wife was the one who was sick. Why was I the one in the hospital? My doctors blamed COPD (chronic obstructive pulmonary disease, a progressive lung disease), asthma, excess fluid in my upper chest, sleep apnea, and even a rare type of high blood pressure that affects arteries in the lungs and in the heart. Or maybe it was a combination of sheer exhaustion, acute anxiety, depression, and grieving.

No doubt about it, I was breaking down physically and emotionally. Would I ever learn to protect my own health? Yes, I wanted to take care of my wife, but I didn't want to be a dead hero. So, in December 2011, I finally contacted the Alzheimer's Association for help. Through the association, I met another Alzheimer's caregiver who became my mentor. He told me he'd had a heart attack, despite having no history of heart disease. That was all the wake-up call I needed. At long last, I was open to using the association's resources and suggestions.

What I Wish I'd Done

I should have started earlier to search out an adult day care so that I could reclaim part of the day for myself, including time for exercise.

Everyone is familiar with the concept of an adrenaline rush, a burst of energy that we associate with a startling, fight-or-flight event. It turns out that other hormones also are released into the body in stressful situations. One of these is cortisol. It was useful to cavemen who had to outrun an attacking animal. But in our modern world, we rarely need that extra spurt of energy, and often it works against our survival. When we live with constant stress, cortisol keeps flooding into our bodies. Without physical activity or other stress busters, the levels stay high and wreak all sorts of havoc. According to the Mayo Clinic, stress is linked to heart disease, mental illnesses, digestive problems, sleep problems, weight gain, and—here's the ironic one for Alzheimer's caregivers—memory and concentration impairment.[11] I've heard some health experts call chronic high stress a ticking time bomb. At least now I know my enemy's name: cortisol.

Here's some more science. A team at Ohio State University and the National Institute on Aging (NIA) spent nearly three decades investigating the links between psychological stress and a weakened immune system. The study, released in 2007, was much more than a survey. It included a comparison of blood samples of Alzheimer's caregivers to those of non-caregivers that revealed a difference at the genetic and molecular level. The scientists concluded that the chronic stress of Alzheimer's caregiving may shorten spouses' and children's lives by as much as four to eight years.[12] Think about that: that's four to eight years you won't see your grandkids grow up.

The Mayo Clinic, Ohio State University, and the NIA aren't alone in looking at the possible links between Alzheimer's and caregiver health. It's certainly a hot topic for anyone interested in health-care reform and holding down expenditures. Back in 2010, economist Brent Fulton from the University of California, Berkeley, determined that Alzheimer's caregivers spend 8 percent more on health care than non-caregivers. In a more recent estimate, the Alzheimer's Association calculated that in 2018, the physical and emotional impact of dementia caregiving in the United States resulted in an estimated $11.8 billion—again, billion with a *b*—in health-care costs.[13]

As the research continues to reveal the unfortunate implications for the health of Alzheimer's caregivers, you continue to climb the Alzheimer's mountain.

To me, being an Alzheimer's caregiver is like being the fictional boxer Rocky Balboa in a pitched battle against a much stronger opponent. The disease can back you into a corner. You have to maintain your footing as you swing away. You're trying your damnedest to fight back while also struggling to control your own emotions. At the same time, you're absorbing some awful body blows like depression, anxiety, and grief. Each time there's another indication that your partner's mind is being affected, it's another blow.

Unlike Rocky, you'll never be able to defeat your opponent—at least, not when that opponent is Alzheimer's. And if you're not careful, those blows, bit by bit, will defeat you in the trying. Work to understand the illness, and get the help and support you need to respond to it. That's the best path up the mountain.

[Marty] is on the phone with his office again. He does seem to miss the hustle and bustle of work more than enjoying everything here. I'm feeling he is not happy here and is needing more company than just me. I've convinced myself it is just the way it'll have to be. I'm happier here than at home, but I can tell he is missing his workplace and probably his friends there.

—ELAINE'S FLORIDA JOURNAL,
MARCH 28, 2012

CHAPTER 4

⎯⎯⎯ ❧ ⎯⎯⎯

Isolation

M OST PEOPLE PROBABLY THINK of Wisconsin as a terribly cold place. Tune in to a Green Bay Packers game in December (or, hopefully, a home playoff game in January), and you'll see faithful fans bundled up in their snowmobile suits and parkas. Every time those eighty thousand fans exhale or shout their encouragement to their beloved team, you can see their breath. The stadium takes on an eerie energy as the breath vapors appear and then disappear into the cold air.

Cheesehead though I may be, I've also found that I can relate to a different kind of pack than the kind bearing Super Bowl rings: a wolf pack. I once saw a documentary about wolves and it mentioned the way wolf packs will drive out one of their own when resources are scarce. Or sometimes a wolf at the bottom of the pecking order may feel forced to leave the pack for the sake of their own survival. Either way, by exile or by choice, we're left with a lone wolf.

WHEN YOUR PARTNER HAS Alzheimer's, you can feel like that lone wolf, isolated from anyone who cares about your well-being.

If you have joint-replacement surgery or experience cancer (and I've done both), people respond to your immediate needs with understanding and empathy—and food—for the six weeks or six months that you're out of commission. Those acts of kindness are priceless. They fuel your physical healing and feed your spirit. If you're lucky, you reach the end of your rehab or chemo, and then you're able to do things for yourself again. You write thank-you notes, and everyone moves on.

I'd like to think that the weight gained during my early caregiving years resulted from friends and neighbors showering us with rich, home-delivered meals and decadent peach pies. But I'd be kidding myself. Alzheimer's is not a tuna-casserole disease. It's a years-long illness, traumatic for both the person with the disease and the caregiver, with no happy ending this side of heaven.

People don't usually think of offering rides or meals or help with the yard work to an Alzheimer's caregiver. Part of that is because when you're a caregiver, you don't interact with the outside world as much as you used to. Alzheimer's separates you from people you work with, play cards with, attend ball games with, worship with—or, I should say, the people you used to do those things with before caregiving took over your life. They still love you, but they simply don't know how to respond.

Feeling so lonesome was something I didn't anticipate. Like other negative aspects of caregiving, it silently creeps in on you. Caregivers, here is your warning: *loneliness is coming your way.* Its cousin, depression, might show up on your doorstep too.

Many people feel lonely occasionally. In one survey, over 40 percent of people aged sixty-five and older reported being lonely, at least sometimes.[1] What do you suppose the figure is for Alzheimer's caregivers? I'm guessing 100 percent.

Loneliness itself isn't a new topic of interest in the field of psychology. In 1978, researchers at UCLA first developed a twenty-item survey to determine a person's level of loneliness. It's still used today. Unlike the cognitive tests that help diagnose dementia, this test is self-administered. It asks, for example, how often you feel as if no one understands you and how often you feel isolated from other people.[2] Does it make you feel any better if a quickie quiz tells you that you're lonely? Probably not.

Scientists and psychologists have done many studies on loneliness in recent years, and what they're learning is that loneliness is downright dangerous. In a University of Chicago study, lonelier people reported worse physical health, experienced more chronic diseases, and were more likely to develop coronary heart disease.[3] Other research has linked loneliness to problems such as eating disorders, substance abuse, and suicide.[4] Yet another study from researchers at Brigham Young University concluded that loneliness is more harmful than obesity and damages as much as smoking fifteen cigarettes a day.[5]

Loneliness is always a negative experience, according to Rose Beeson, a leading researcher on people who care for a spouse who has Alzheimer's.[6] No kidding.

Heading off loneliness is a two-way street. You can't just put on a brave face day after day. You need to reach out to others and teach them about Alzheimer's. You can't be afraid of sounding like a whiner. To survive, you can't worry that you're being a burden.

And people need to reach out to you. They need to recognize how they can contribute to your well-being with those concrete offers of help.

In the early stages of Elaine's diagnosis, many people didn't know how to respond to our situation because she didn't look sick. They couldn't see what was causing the problem, that her brain was broken. She was struggling to make sense of the world. I didn't look sick, either, but I was suffering from a broken heart as I struggled to accept this awful new reality.

What I Wish I'd Known

The fact that family and friends can't fully understand what a caregiver is going through is not a good enough reason to avoid them.

I did try to keep things somewhat normal as the disease progressed. We had four or five couples with whom we often went out to dinner, and we did for two or three years after Elaine was diagnosed, until she could no longer join in table talk about happenings around town or current events. It became painful to watch her try to fit into social situations. Putting her in a position where she had to carry on a coherent conversation was as cruel as challenging someone on crutches to a tennis match.

For the next five or six years, the two of us did dine out a lot—for probably 90 percent of our meals—because even with my help Elaine couldn't so much as boil water (and I'm not much of a cook myself). She was always right across the table from me, yet those restaurant meals became increasingly sad experiences for me.

At home there wasn't much to talk about either. Earlier in the disease, Elaine had to resign from the boards of several organizations around town because she really couldn't participate in their activities. By the time she was in the middle stages of the disease (about five years after her diagnosis), she had lost all interest in reading, making photo albums, shopping, baking, and so many other things she used to enjoy. She was anxious and bored.

Two of our four children live far from Milwaukee, several states away. Certainly, I kept all of them in the loop. But I didn't think it was helpful to overdramatize the situation. You say, "Alzheimer's," and that's enough for your kids to understand the importance of spending time with Mom before she slips away completely. Each of them has handled the situation differently, and I can't say any of them has gotten it wrong.

The kids try their best to keep the connection with their mother alive. Naturally, it has become tougher as time passes. When you speak to someone face-to-face (whether they have dementia or not), eye contact and gestures communicate so much; of course, those things are missing over the phone. As Alzheimer's tightened its grip on Elaine's brain, she would repeat questions to the kids ("How are you?" "How is your family?") sometimes five or six times. Ever hear someone say, "It's good just to hear your voice"? In this case, the voice was familiar, but Elaine's limited vocabulary was a painful reminder to our children that she was dying mentally. The kids' calls became shorter and less frequent, and I can't blame them. Why call and have a continued painful experience?

My professional relationships were affected too. Over the decades, I had worn out several sets of tires making the 160-mile round trip to the Wisconsin State Capitol in Madison for various meetings and events. But now, I had no desire to work with members of the Wisconsin State Legislature—Republican or Democrat—on issues I should have cared about. I felt much better withdrawn than being involved. I was just too exhausted to go and too content staying home.

I didn't even budge during election season (which practically never ends in a battleground state like Wisconsin). Important people are always coming here for rallies and fundraisers. Had I wanted to, I could have shared the stage with all sorts of Democratic Party dignitaries, including presidential and vice-presidential candidates. Government is in my blood. For me to step away from the political arena was like a compulsive shopper staying home on Black Friday.

And remember all the skipped workouts that contributed to my health problems? Besides the exercise I missed out on, I was giving up my social interactions with that group of friends as well.

What I Wish I'd Done

I should have worked to find a healthy outlet for my own sadness and fearfulness so that anticipatory grief wouldn't limit my day-to-day functioning.

What I needed was someone to talk to about Alzheimer's. I needed someone to at least acknowledge the pain I was experiencing.

What I also needed was to *not* talk about Alzheimer's. I needed activities that focused my energy on my own interests and needs.

I needed to break the cycle of isolation that was eating me alive.

One other thing I needed: the ability to deal with mounting stress.

Marty is still a very good husband, and I can't blame him for being a little short sometimes. [My disease] has to be a problem for him. It puts more responsibility [on him] than he can handle sometimes. But he knows I'm trying my best, and he tries hard to help me. I know it is no easier for him than for me.

—Elaine's notes during a visit to
Door County, Wisconsin, July 3, 2012

CHAPTER 5

——⚭——

Irrational Irritability

Even though Alzheimer's was causing Elaine to behave erratically, in 2011, I decided we should go visit our daughter Kathy, who lives near Boston. When it came time to leave the hotel room, I discovered that, sometime while my back was turned, Elaine had unpacked all the luggage and returned items to the dresser drawers. She had done that at home before a trip, thinking she was being helpful. But now? When we needed to get to Logan International? Now the race was on to find and re-pack everything and make it to the airport on time. With the clock ticking, our taxi raced to Logan. Almost miraculously, we got through security and to our gate just before they closed the door to the jetway.

We were the last people to board the plane and our two seats were the only ones left—at the back, of course. I trudged down the aisle with Elaine following, relieved we'd made it but out of breath, each of us dragging a suitcase. Does it surprise you to learn that I couldn't get the bags to fit under the seat and the overhead bins were full?

I asked the flight attendant what to do with our bags.

"You know," she replied, "we wouldn't have this trouble if you weren't the last people on the airplane."

Well, that lit my fuse! The anger welling up inside me came out as almost hatred. After all I had gone through to get us there on time, all this flight attendant could suggest was that we should have arrived earlier? Couldn't she see that I was desperately trying to catch my breath? "This has got to be," I declared, "the world's worst goddamn airline."

With that, the flight attendant rushed to the front of the plane to talk to her coworkers. As they looked back at me, I was sure they were discussing whether I was a threat to their safety and should be taken off the plane.

I LIKE TO THINK of myself as a pretty even-keeled guy. You have to have a thick skin to be in politics; it doesn't pay to get worked up about every little thing. My company's website brags about my charm and wit—hey, it's on the internet, so it must be true, right?

Charm and wit did not do me one iota of good on another trip, this time to Florida in November 2012. We planned to vacation there for the winter to escape the Wisconsin weather, so I took along cash to cover some meals and other expenses. A thousand dollars. It wasn't my best decision ever, but I put the cash in a jar on the dresser. The next day, it was gone. "Elaine, where is that money? Did you take that money?" For all I knew, she had flushed it down the toilet. A thousand dollars! Frantic and furious, I searched for those fifty- and one-hundred-dollar bills everywhere. Buckets of cortisol must have been coursing through my body. Thankfully, four days later, I found the cash—stuffed into a sock in the dresser. It must have been Elaine's way of hiding it safely away, once again trying to demonstrate that she could help. She had no idea of the consequences of her action.

What I Wish I'd Known

Unfamiliar settings such as hotels can be particularly upsetting to people with dementia because they have trouble reorienting.

Honestly, I should have known better. Starting two or three years before this incident, I would find checks and cash stowed away in drawers and clothing all over our home in Milwaukee. When those things began happening, I took over all the management of our finances to keep things straight. It was not only one more thing I had to tackle but also sad for me because Elaine had always handled all that so well—banking, credit cards, investing, charitable giving, the whole nine yards. As the disease took its toll, I was terrified that she might give away our life savings to telephone solicitors; thankfully, she didn't. One task she remained very good at was ordering packs of checks from our credit union—I found boxes with hundreds of newly printed checks. Looking on the bright side, that should cover us for a few years!

One more lost-item story: Once, Elaine put the car keys in the dishwasher. So the next time I couldn't find the keys, I assumed her helpful behavior was the explanation—she must have put them in her idea of a safe place—and I figured the next two hours of my life would be spent searching for those damn keys. (Yes, I did check the dishwasher, without success. People with Alzheimer's don't often put things away in the same place.) The blame game was already underway. This tale has a happy ending though with a twist. I learned it's best not to accuse your wife of hiding the car keys until you've checked your own coat pockets.

Something as big as nearly missing your flight or something as small as misplaced car keys gets magnified when you are an Alzheimer's caregiver. You are trying to do so much, and at the same time, you're dealing with sadness and grieving. Your instinct is to multitask your to-do list to death. If doing more than one thing at a time is something you can manage, all well and good. The risk comes in overloading yourself. When you can't give something your full attention, often the result is that you get less done, not more. That makes you tired, resentful, and crabby—a Grumpy Old Man, as it were.

I call this phenomenon "irrational irritability." You probably remember this emotion from those sleep-deprived days when your children were babies. Fortunately for parents, it's a lot easier to bounce back when you're in your twenties, thirties, or forties. And at least you know the sleepless nights aren't going to last forever.

An exhausted, stressed-out Alzheimer's caregiver who is sixty, seventy, or eighty years old, meanwhile, has a different threshold of anxiety. You get to the end of your rope quicker. Things that really shouldn't bother you, really do! This can lead to making poor decisions or saying hurtful things that you instantly regret. The last thing you want to do is drive people away, but it can easily happen. You don't want to know how many bouquets of flowers and boxes of candy I have given to friends, relatives, and even store clerks as peace offerings after losing my cool. Although I still believe that Boston flight attendant could have been far more helpful, maybe I should have sent flowers to her too.

Sadly, some caregivers even lash out at their loved ones with dementia. Elder abuse has been a concern of mine going back to the early 1970s when, as lieutenant governor, I led a task force on overhauling Wisconsin's nursing home licensing and regulating system. Mistreatment of people who live in care facilities is a disgusting crime, and it goes on despite state and federal abuse-prevention laws—not to mention decency and common sense.

What I'm talking about here, though, is abuse and neglect by family members. Various studies report that up to 90 percent of those who abuse the elderly are family members.[1] Researchers have also found that family members who abuse drugs and/or alcohol, who have a mental and/or emotional illness, and who feel burdened by their caregiving responsibilities abuse at higher rates than those who are not in such situations.[2]

When it comes to people with dementia, nearly half of their family caregivers (47.3 percent) were abusive, according to a study published in the *Journal of the American Geriatrics Society*.[3] Verbal mistreatment by caregivers is the most reported type of abuse, at 60 percent . Next comes neglect at 14 percent. And, unfortunately, 5 to 10 percent of caregivers are physically abusive toward a person with dementia.[4]

Obviously, it's difficult to come up with accurate statistics because care recipients may be unable to talk about any abuse that is taking place and caregivers may not be truthful in answering questions about abusive behavior. But there is no question in my mind that family caregivers sometimes abuse those with Alzheimer's or another form of dementia. We get irritable and sometimes behave irrationally. People who are hurting, hurt people.

And you are hurting. As your spouse's Alzheimer's progresses, you will face conversations that break your heart. You can't take it personally when your loved one can't remember names and events. When your curious, charming, four-year-old grandchild asks, "Why?" over and over, sure, it can get old. But when it's an adult yanking your chain (even though it's the disease talking), frustration is a natural reaction. Ask any caregiver if he or she ever feels like screaming, and if the person is being honest, the answer will be, "Yes, and I not only feel like it—I have screamed!"

It's a very human thing to feel trapped and hopeless. Under stress and trying to adjust to—and accept—your new reality, it's easy to pick at that scab. You flip your lid over something that would never bother you under normal circumstances. Of course you are angry. But be angry at the disease and not at your loved one. To direct anger at your loved one is extremely harmful, not to mention unproductive, foolish, and inappropriate. If you feel yourself teetering on the edge of emotional or physical harm, make sure to get help immediately. It may be necessary to do more than simply count to ten and walk away for a minute. Do whatever it takes to deal with your emotions.

To be the best—and most patient—caregiver possible, you need the right approach. It starts, as I explained in chapter 1, with recognizing that Alzheimer's is an enemy you cannot defeat. It continues, as I told you in chapter 3, with protecting your own health. And it requires new strategies, such as perhaps putting your suitcases into the trunk of the car right after you pack them.

It also takes letting go of being in control (more on that in chapter 7). No one says you have to care alone.

What I Wish I'd Done

I should have paid more attention to reducing my stress so that I wouldn't become irrationally irritable, distracted, and forgetful.

I'll admit that, starting on this climb about eighteen years ago, I didn't know what Alzheimer's really was, how it would impact our lives, and how ill-equipped I was to take on the role of caregiver. Elaine and I were only in our mid-sixties when she began showing symptoms of cognitive impairment. We had expected to have many happy years to look forward to, but they were taken away from us. I felt cheated. I stubbornly held on to the Elaine that once was. I didn't always accept the obvious new normal, such as the need to give myself enough time to get the job done—and maybe redone, if my wife unpacked my suitcase—so I could head off a meltdown. I didn't enjoy losing control of my emotions. Every time I blew up, I swore it would be the last time. If you were ever a victim of my irrational irritability, I apologize that you were the casualty of my hurt.

The resources and support of my local Alzheimer's Association chapter helped me finally pull it together. They nudged me into sharing my story in very public ways, such as this book, and that has helped me find a purpose in life. I hope my message is getting through to you so you can be an effective caregiver who learns, copes, and survives.

PART 2

Coping with
Alzheimer's Disease

[I am] not enjoying my role any more as Marty's wife. Because of his having concerns about my Alzheimer's, he doesn't let me be me. [I can't] go for a walk if I want to, or to the store alone, etc., etc. I used to appreciate him—what I thought was concern—but he holds me captive much too much. I am going to try to have a second opinion because I really don't think I have any problem. I know how to drive or walk anyplace I want to enjoy, but he doesn't believe me, and I hate the control he has placed on me. I don't even think I have Alzheimer's per se.

—ELAINE'S JOURNAL, 2009

CHAPTER 6

Reaching for a Lifeline

A WOMAN HAD A parrot. All day long, for hours, for years, the parrot would repeat, "Polly wants a party. Polly wants a party." The woman was expecting some important company and became concerned about the image she would project if her parrot squawked, "Polly wants a party. Polly wants a party," while she entertained her distinguished guests.

At her wit's end, the woman went to her priest to ask for advice. The good father could hardly believe the coincidence—he himself had two parrots, Peter Parrot and Paul Parrot. What was so special about these birds, he explained, was that for many years his parrots had fervently prayed. They prayed from morning to night, every waking hour.

The priest suggested that the woman bring Polly to the church to meet Peter and Paul. He was sure his pious parrots would provide the powerful, positive influence that Polly so obviously needed.

With great hope, the woman hurried home and retrieved Polly. Predictably, as soon as the parrot was put into the cage with the priest's birds, she loudly screeched, "Polly wants a party. Polly wants a party."

With that, Peter Parrot looked at Paul Parrot and said, "Our prayers have finally been answered!"

FINDING THE RIGHT WAY to provide for Elaine's changing needs over our climb up this Alzheimer's mountain has required persistence and determination, the likes of which I did not know I could muster.

Long before I recognized that I needed help as a caregiver, Elaine and I were working together to find the best ways to maintain her quality of life. As I mentioned earlier, when she first was diagnosed in 2007, she devoted her energy to reading all she could about Alzheimer's. We stayed busy with walks and time with friends. That was not enough.

Through her own research, Elaine affirmed how important it was to exercise. That led to her identifying a nearby community center that had an indoor pool. Elaine thought this would be an ideal way to stay in good physical shape and do something positive for herself. You didn't even have to sign up for a membership—just pay as you go—so there was no pressure. Elaine, who had been a lifelong swimmer, soon was going there three mornings a week and making friends. The center also offered massage therapy, including Reiki. Elaine had read that massage helped both the body and the mind relax, so she added that to her schedule once a week. She even drove herself there; after all, it was barely three minutes from home.

For several months, it really was perfect. Unfortunately, her symptoms were gradually getting worse.

That's how Alzheimer's is. You think you have this thing figured out, and then you don't.

A symptom that began to take hold of Elaine was excessive shopping. To support its many programs, the community center operated a sort of thrift store and gift shop. Costume jewelry, shirts, skirts, blouses, sweaters, glassware, books, movies, candle holders, even eight-track tapes all began finding their way into our home. She never came home empty-handed! It took me a while to understand why all this buying was so important to her. I concluded that she thought she had to do her part to help this community center succeed. Since then, I learned that hoarding is one of the behaviors people with dementia might exhibit; experts say it can stem from the person's fear that they may need the items someday.

Around this time, the bigger problem for Elaine was that driving was increasingly more difficult. Even though the pool was only a mile and a half down the street, she was getting lost. This upset her and was obviously unsafe for her as well as anyone else on the road. Fortunately, she was able to continue going to the center for a while, thanks to a neighbor who provided her rides; sometimes I drove her too.

As I waited for her at the center, I learned that it also offered adult day services and a specialized program for people with dementia. Elaine might not have needed five-days-a-week services, but I thought that a couple of days might benefit us both. Staff members saw that I was suffering from shortness of breath and told me of their concern. The social worker could tell that my spirit was suffering too. It was obvious to them that I needed some more "me" time, more than the hour I got during Elaine's swim or massage.

What the outside world didn't see was that I was beginning to lean more and more on what I call the "caregivers' poison"—alcohol—to cope with my sad situation. I would reach five in the afternoon and consider myself successful for having made it through another day as a caregiver. I wasn't brimming with pride; I was just relieved and thinking that maybe my worries were behind me for a few hours. Time to relax with a drink or two.

It was, in a way, comforting. The alcohol not only numbed my mind but also helped me escape reality. I felt calmer, more at ease. My evenings were not marked by the irrational irritability that caused me so much trouble at times during the day. Drinking also enabled me to fall asleep quite easily. Although once the alcohol wore off during the night, it was back to awake awareness and restless nights of interrupted sleep.

The reality is that all the armies marching and all the navies sailing cannot, at this time, stop Alzheimer's. Likewise, drinking all the beer brewed and all the whiskey aged cannot change the course of this disease. Alcohol use can be the caregiver's curse. It has to be recognized and dealt with. Otherwise, there is one more monster—quite an ugly one at that—to make life more difficult for both the caregiver and the person with dementia.

I was fortunate in that I was a "short hitter." Plus, our daughter Kristine was tuned in to the situation and talked with me about it. She also provided me an article on the benefits of moderate drinking; be assured that it was not given to me because I was drinking too little. My doctor became concerned as well and told me I was over self-medicating, to put it politely. (I still work to limit my drinks to two a day. Most times I succeed.)

With all this playing in the background, I wanted Elaine to at least try a day program so I could get some respite.

This could have been our turning point. But Elaine would have no part of it.

Sadly, we left that community center, and whatever help it could have offered, a few months later when swimming no longer was a suitable activity for Elaine. We were on our own again.

I thought the answer to our situation might be to bring help into our home. I contacted a home care agency. That was tricky because Elaine was adamantly opposed to any professional caregivers invading her turf. Women like my wife can be protective of their kitchens, and people with Alzheimer's can have an even more difficult time with someone else being in their home. They can be distrustful of strangers and even of friends and family. They may even accuse people of stealing, which partially explains why people with dementia tend to move (hide) valuables.

The first couple of in-home helpers suggested by the agency were younger women. That really made Elaine uncomfortable. I tried someone more her age, but that was no better. Not to be easily defeated, I kept trying. I attempted to explain to Elaine that the home care wasn't for her, saying it was for me, but she told me, "That's your problem." So next, I tried lying (more on that in chapter 8). I made up a story that this lady (actually the caregiver) was new in town. She wanted someone to walk her around the neighborhood and show her where different businesses, parks, and churches were and to help her find her way around a new grocery store. I thought that was pretty clever. Whether or not Elaine saw through my story, it didn't succeed. She declared that this new-lady-in-town's difficulties were not her responsibility. This defiant attitude was in sharp contrast to Elaine's usually gracious personality.

All told, the community center experience and my attempts to have care provided for Elaine in our home consumed more than a year after her diagnosis. Obviously, Elaine's symptoms were getting worse. I still had not accessed caregiver support of any kind; my focus was on what would benefit Elaine. I started looking for another option.

What I Wish I'd Known

The Alzheimer's Association and AARP offer a comprehensive search tool with information on local programs and care centers. Go to https://www .communityresourcefinder.org.

I'd heard that a care facility in town offered an adult day-care program for people in the early stages of memory loss, and I thought it was worth checking out. Elaine already was familiar with this facility because her mother had spent the final years of her life there. Fortunately, Elaine was agreeable to going one day a week to what we called "continuing education." By the grace of God, she did not associate this program with dementia care.

Elaine was "going to classes " and indeed dutifully took a college-ruled notebook with her and made use of it every week. The staff and volunteers helped small groups of participants play games and do memory exercises. Elaine became almost obsessed with journaling every part of the experience. One time, the group went on a field trip to a candy factory in a town about an hour away. Her notebook covered the bus ride in remarkable detail, with highlights of many street corners and nearly exact turn-by-turn directions.

Elaine also kept a journal when we were in Florida over the winter of 2011 to 2012. By then she got her days mixed up easily. I did my best to help her keep things straight, but I didn't always have time for her questions because I was busy on my laptop or phone, tending to business matters back home. So, I bought her a special digital clock that clearly displayed the date and day of the week as well as the time. She also referred to the newspaper each day to help her keep track of the calendar. A byproduct of that routine was that she was well aware of the upcoming presidential election—she mentioned it over and over in her vacation journal, the cover of which featured a whimsical scene of several dogs seated on porch chairs overlooking the beach.

But before we traveled to Florida in 2011, something quite significant had happened that fall.

Although I was convinced that we already had gone to enough doctors—there had been at least four since 2005—Elaine wanted to be seen by a woman doctor. Completely on her own, without my knowledge, she made a call to the 24-7 Alzheimer's Association helpline (1-800-272-3900) in search of a suggestion. Meanwhile, in another part of the association's southeastern Wisconsin offices, work was well underway to plan the annual Walk to End Alzheimer's. At that time, one of the walk's organizers told the staff that she desperately needed a person with early stage dementia to speak at the fundraiser because the original speaker had just canceled. With Elaine's permission, the helpline counselor shared her first name with the walk organizer, who then contacted Elaine. In that conversation, Elaine disclosed that she was Elaine Schreiber, the former first lady of Wisconsin. When asked to participate, Elaine told the organizer, "I will be a public face of this disease," and within a week, she was appearing on local TV to promote the walk.

On the cool, sunshiny day of the walk, Elaine wore an official purple T-shirt, a red baseball cap, and the biggest, friendliest smile you can imagine. She proudly stood onstage to show the world that a person with early-stage Alzheimer's looks like anybody else. When she took the microphone, she thanked the participants for coming and urged them to get involved with the association. Her remarks were brief and well-delivered; as you might expect, she had written them out in advance. A college campus, a crowd of thousands, let's-get-fired-up music over the loudspeaker—the event had all the trappings of a political rally, only this time it was Elaine who was the center of attention.

By reaching out, Elaine had not only received the referral she sought but also made herself known to the association. An invaluable relationship was established. Lines of communication were opened that began to change our lives. It is no exaggeration to describe Elaine's initial phone call to the helpline as monumental and transformative.

A year later in October 2012, we were back at the Walk to End Alzheimer's with my firm's name printed on the back of the T-shirts as a sponsor.

Before we returned to Florida in November 2012, our dear friends Don and Karen, who lived in the vacation condo next door to ours, had researched adult-care programs in the area. They even visited four or five places before we arrived; they helped me choose a program that would meet Elaine's needs. If you can believe our good fortune, it was located only about a mile away and was operated by a Lutheran church.

What I Wish I'd Done

From the beginning, I should have shared more information about Elaine and concerns about my ability to cope so that I could have begun to focus on surviving.

By the time we came back to Wisconsin in April 2013, Elaine was so accustomed to attending "classes" that she was ready for a program that met every weekday. Together, we toured a facility near downtown Milwaukee and met with several staff members.

They were positive, smiling, and courteous. It's a good thing Elaine was so willing to go there. Even after a winter in the warm Florida sun, I was more and more in need of respite time.

Five mornings a week, she'd fuss with her hair and makeup before we headed to breakfast. She was armed with her spiral notebook when I took her to "class" for the day, usually around 9:00 a.m. I would pick her up at 3:00 or 3:30 in the afternoon.

I wish I could say that the weekday program put an end to my daily stress. It did buy me a few hours to do some household chores, maybe get in some exercise or tackle some of my company's work that had been pushed off to the side for so long. The problem was the black cloud of Alzheimer's that followed me everywhere. My mind remained busy with thoughts of what the disease was doing to Elaine and what surely was coming. There was a growing and unavoidable sense of foreboding.

I wish my Alzheimer's would dissipate. I'd like to be the smart wife and mother I used to be. Now, I have to waste so much time just trying to figure out what I should be doing—without seeming as smart as I used to be. I need to rely on Marty for everything. And I'm very lucky he continues to keep me. Life gets more difficult every day.

—A NOTE BY ELAINE, DATE UNKNOWN

CHAPTER 7

―∞―

Being a Real Man

A FTER I LOST THE race for governor in 1978, we moved to a
hobby farm in central Wisconsin. I had always loved horses
as a child. Man, how I lived for the one-hour-a-year horseback
ride my parents would treat me to at the Kettle Moraine State
Forest, an hour from Milwaukee. So, this move was my chance
to buy a horse. Her name was Brianna, but for the purpose of this
story–to make it more exciting–I will use the name Thunderbolt Killer.

I got a great bargain when I bought this mare since she wasn't
fully broken to the saddle. I hired a trainer to help me every Saturday morning. Between sessions, I'd work on the skills we had
learned, before something new was introduced. One Saturday,
the trainer took a rope and tied one end to the halter on the
horse's head and the other to the horse's tail–she was connected
to herself in a sort of turned position. Thunderbolt Killer just
stood there. "This is one smart horse," the trainer said. "Most
horses would buck and jump, but you've got one that's first trying to figure out how it got into this predicament and how to get
out of it."

71

WITH ALZHEIMER'S CAREGIVING, THERE'S no point in bucking and jumping whenever you find yourself in a difficult situation. That only creates more havoc. You need to be smart. *How did I get into this predicament, and how am I going to untangle myself safely?* The answer is: it didn't happen overnight, and you're going to need a lot of help.

Though what follows can also apply to wives taking care of their husbands, the shift in roles is often more challenging for men who become caregivers—so I will speak very bluntly to you husbands in this chapter. You and your wife have always been a team, building each other's careers and sharing in the work of raising a family. Now, the balance will shift little by little until you'll be taking care of her a lot more than she takes care of you. You'll do all the driving. You'll go to all her doctor appointments and manage her medications. You'll take over the housework, shopping, and cooking. You'll choose her clothing and help her get dressed. You'll help her safely take a shower and, eventually, even help her use the toilet.

You'll do all that—and much more—with a broken heart. I know that your instinct is to try carrying this weight alone. Being a "real man" means being brave, suffering in silence, and standing on your own two feet, right? You're not supposed to depend on others, are you? There's a lot of truth in the old stereotype that male drivers don't like to stop and ask for directions. But to be a good caregiver, asking for help is exactly what you have to do. That's how you show how strong you are.

Before Alzheimer's, I'd spent a lifetime in politics and business delegating responsibility to my staff and employees. Somehow, dealing with this disease was different. For many months, I wasn't very public about Elaine's diagnosis and how I was being impacted. I guess I didn't want to unload on people beyond the circle of our closest friends. Stubborn, stupid Marty!

There's no shame in your spouse having Alzheimer's, and there's no shame in your asking for help. And if I had spent time in a support group sooner, I'd have known that sooner.

When I finally did reach out to the Alzheimer's Association, about four years into my climb up this caregiving mountain, I began meeting with a counselor at my local chapter's office. She put me in contact with other caregivers, whom I found easy to talk to one-on-one. Collectively, they helped me understand that you can't go it alone.

Did you catch that? It took me *four years* to begin working with the Alzheimer's Association to get the help I needed. During those four years, I had health problems that possibly could have been avoided. I don't want you to wait anywhere near that long to take advantage of the association's support.

I know I am repeating myself, but I feel I have to do that because my message is so important: get help. Take out your phone right now and add the helpline number for the Alzheimer's Association (1-800-272-3900) into your contacts list. Remember: it's a free, 24-7 resource that offers information about the disease, treatment options, caregiver skills, and much more.

What I Wish I'd Known

Asking others to help does not mean you're not strong enough or not trying hard enough.

When it comes to having someone to turn to, let's face it: most men don't have as many close friends as women do. But whether man or woman, if you are the primary caregiver for a person with dementia, take a minute right now and name three people outside your family in whom you can confide.

This isn't like Facebook where you might have hundreds of "friends." I'm talking about the true-blue friends who will listen long enough to know what it's really like to be married to someone who has Alzheimer's. Even if your list is three people—or especially if you can't come up with that many—you need to reach out to the Alzheimer's Association. They'll help you.

One thing that makes it hard to ask friends for help is that Alzheimer's makes most people uncomfortable. Few people understand what it's about; all they know is it's not good. In fairness to my friends, they, too, are grieving the loss of the First Elaine. For the longest time, I was satisfied just to have a friend ask, "What can I do?" The offer itself was comforting. You might even say it's like having a million dollars in the bank. But that million-dollar account doesn't mean anything if you don't spend fifty bucks now and then.

It seems obvious, but every hour not spent on errands or chores is time you have for other things—whether it's something your spouse needs or taking better care of yourself. What's on your to-do list? Could someone else buy a few groceries this week? Drop off dry-cleaning? Return library books? Walk the dog? Run your car through the car wash? Or bring you a tuna casserole?

With a better comprehension of how Alzheimer's was affecting Elaine, I would have known what kind of help to ask for. For example, when Elaine was in the early stages of the disease, I could have requested that a friend take her for a walk or out for coffee. She usually did better in one-on-one situations where little was expected of her. I enjoyed those times, and I bet her friends would have too.

What I Wish I'd Done

I should have enlisted a couple of friends to be my team captains, who could do the asking and scheduling for me.

And I could have had some respite time when our children visited from out of town. They certainly were willing to help. But I still considered their visits to be occasions to entertain them and take care of them as Elaine and I had done for the previous twenty years. What I really needed, however, was to rest. It wasn't until I was beyond physically worn out that I finally allowed myself the luxury to sleep in or grab a nap while they were here to help with Elaine. I shouldn't have pretended for so long that I was doing fine.

There are lots of ways to recruit and organize your helpers. You can set up a personalized schedule online or via a smartphone app. Such a calendar lets you list what kind of help you need and when, and friends can sign up to pitch in. Some specific resources include CareCalendar, CaringBridge, Caring Village, or Lotsa Helping Hands. On SignUpGenius, you can set up a calendar so volunteers can bring meals.

Be sure you have current email addresses and phone numbers for people who might be able to help. Send out a group message ("Dear friends, please excuse my manners in not asking you face-to-face, but I am having a difficult time managing all the things I need to do ..."). If technology isn't your thing, see if a friend will organize a phone tree or mail out a letter to some of your friends. As the word gets around, I know you will get offers of help.

For the first four years—four long years—as I hiked the Alzheimer's trail, I stuck to my crazy notion that I didn't need anyone's map or suggestions. I believed that as long as I loved Elaine (and

I'd had a half century of practice at that already), I could handle the rest. Thank heaven I finally realized how wrong I had been. Look at what my attitude cost me—aggravation, good health, lost moments of joy with Elaine, and a friend or two along the way. Caregiver burnout and loneliness feed on each other. Admit you need help. Then get it.

Everyone but [Marty] tells me how well I'm doing and [I]
always hear I should continue doing everything I have
been—as most of my friends tell me I am doing well and if
they didn't know I had Alzheimer's wouldn't know. I, too,
feel that I am as normal as most people in their seventies.

—ELAINE'S NOTES DURING A VISIT TO
DOOR COUNTY, WISCONSIN, JULY 3, 2012

CHAPTER 8

Therapeutic Fibbing:
Entering Her Reality

A MAN IS OUT driving one afternoon and comes across an injured pedestrian in the roadway. He knows that medical care is needed immediately, so he calls 911 and frantically tells the operator, "You've got to send help right away to Pistachio Street."

The operator says, "How do you spell *Pistachio*?"

The man says, "I don't know! What I do know is he needs the EMTs!"

The operator says, "I'm sorry, I can't dispatch the ambulance without inputting the correct street name on my computer."

"Okay," says the man. "I'll call you back in five minutes."

"Five minutes! Why five minutes?" asks the operator.

The man replies, "I'm going to drag the guy a block over to Elm Street."

THE STARK REALITY IS that if your partner ever did know how to spell *pistachio*, he or she won't for long.

Often, when cognitive problems first start to show, you find yourself trying to fill in the gaps, providing a detail your partner is trying to recall or prompting with a word he or she can't come up with. *Old age*, you tell yourself.

Then you find out it's Alzheimer's.

The greater stark reality is that conversations are only going to get more difficult. You might be tempted to jump in more than ever before to fill in the blanks. It takes a lot of patience to hold yourself back and give your partner a chance to make the point, even if he or she is wrong. Know this: you cannot argue with Alzheimer's and expect to win.

Trying to set your spouse straight when he or she gets a detail wrong in some old family story is an exhausting exercise. It can turn into a disagreement that's completely unnecessary. Is it really important that you two went to the seafood place, not the steakhouse, to celebrate your partner's fiftieth birthday?

Your partner may not remember actually having a fiftieth birthday. One time, Elaine asked, "How old am I?" Rather than chiding her for not knowing or even giving her a straight answer, I asked, "How old do you want to be?" And we had a good laugh.

For your own sanity, get rid of the idea that you are always right. Lose the attitude! Do you want to be right, or do you want to be happy? You are now living in two realities: your partner's and yours. Spending time in that Alzheimer's reality is an important way to demonstrate your love.

Neuroscientist Naomi Eisenberger of UCLA—coincidentally, the same university that developed the loneliness scale I mentioned a few chapters ago—conducted studies on images of the brain that have helped researchers conclude that loving relationships alter the brain in positive ways.[1] Essayist Diane Ackerman calls it the brain on love: "When your brain knows you're with someone you can trust, it needn't waste precious resources coping with stressors or menace."[2] Of course, that's not to say that you can love away someone's dementia. We all wish it were that simple.

When you try to reason with someone who has Alzheimer's, it only intensifies the trouble (and activates your stress hormones). You've got to remind yourself that while your partner looks the same on the outside, things are very different on the inside. Dementia is transforming the world into a reality unfamiliar to you. Especially in the late stages of Alzheimer's, a person with dementia is happier in his or her own world. Your job is to keep your partner's mind at ease so he or she feels safe and loved. Alzheimer's caregivers call it "compassionate communication."

There's no good reason to correct Elaine when she thinks I've been in Madison on business all day when in fact I've been in Milwaukee. The truth is out there, as they say, but it isn't important. I join along with her and enjoy the conversation. I might retell a short story about something special that happened when we lived in Madison or just agree with her. "Yes, honey, I was in Madison, and the traffic coming back was a real mess."

This is "therapeutic fibbing." I have to admit, that sounds better than "providing false testimony," as my dusty old law school textbooks would call it. And it's a lot more palatable than "lying," which is what people think politicians do most of the time. Imagine if I'd known this was an option fifty-eight years ago when we were first married, or in my campaigns for governor and mayor!

Getting serious again, I've discovered that little white lies are a means to a more peaceful relationship with someone who has Alzheimer's. I call it therapeutic because it's a tonic that tamps down some of the pain with which you are living.

What I Wish I'd Known

You're a healthier, happier, and more helpful caregiver if you are less confrontational.

Fibbing is a useful tactic when a person with dementia asks about family members and friends. Women and men will always be concerned about the people they love. How is my dad? Is my brother all right? A parent will wonder and worry about his or her children. As the ability to process and remember information diminishes, your job is to deflect your partner's fears and concerns.

"Are our kids doing okay?" you'll be asked—probably over and over.

"Yes, everyone's fine," you'll respond.

I once made the terrible mistake of answering one of Elaine's questions about her parents by telling her the truth, that they were dead. She looked as sad as the day many years earlier when she'd learned that they had died.

"Dead?" she repeated, concerned and puzzled. "Did we take good care of them? Did I go to their funerals?" She was distraught to think that maybe she hadn't honored them properly. What good did it do to give her a real-world answer when she lives in her own altered world? Until I saw the sorrow in her eyes, I didn't know that the truth wasn't always relevant. I vowed I wouldn't put her through that kind of pain again.

Sometime later, we heard a piece of music that made her think of her folks; she remarked that they would enjoy it (present tense). Not that they would have enjoyed it (past tense). This time, I responded in the way I now knew was better for her. "They sure would," I told her.

More recently, with Alzheimer's continuing to squeeze the memory out of Elaine's brain, she told me something odd yet sweet. It was a statement I didn't dare dispute. In fact, I took it as a great compliment. She said, "You look just like my husband."

Another very helpful approach is "redirecting." The idea is to change the focus of the person with dementia, thereby preventing a conversation from turning into an argument. For instance, when Elaine asks me for a glass of wine at 9:00 a.m., there's no point in giving her the dozen reasons why that's not happening. Instead, I shift the discussion to other things related to wine. For instance, I talk about how pretty wine looks in its glass or ask who else she would like to drink wine with. After a few minutes of that, she's moved on. Use your partner's framework (here, the wine) and redirect to another subject (in this case, wine glasses and friends).

What I Wish I'd Done

I should have used my wife's frame of reference instead of challenging it.

Tense situations also can come up because a person with Alzheimer's increasingly has trouble relating to logical boundaries. Dementia can cause someone to pick up things unnecessarily and move them. (You do remember the panic that resulted from the suitcase-unpacking incident and the misplaced-cash fiasco, right?) Or it could be that your partner picks up something that doesn't belong to him or her. Maybe your partner wants to put on someone else's sweater or reaches for the wrong glass at dinner. You can waste time and energy trying to correct your partner, or you can let it go. Ask yourself, *Does it matter? Is anyone at risk of injury?* If others are with you, make sure they understand what is going on, explain the best response in such situations, and advise them to accept this as normal for Alzheimer's. Help them so you all can let it go!

Better yet, thank your partner for "finding" the sweater or glass you've been "looking for." With this response, you not only avoid a confrontation but also give that person an opportunity to feel proud. To feel useful. To hear in your voice and see in your facial expression that you're grateful for the help.

Therapeutic fibbing and redirecting are two of the best ways I've found to keep stress from consuming me (you can read even more tips for employing these strategies in appendix B). They've also given me the opportunity to turn a potential "I'm right, you're wrong" conversation into a moment of joy. It's all part of knowing how Alzheimer's plays out. It's a way to cope.

Life is better than ever. Even my knee is cooperating and Marty too. He's finally relaxing more. We took our morning walk and saw at least ten little lizards along the way. Nature has a way of making you appreciate life— including our wonderful human time together.

—ELAINE'S FLORIDA JOURNAL,
APRIL 5, 2012

CHAPTER 9

Living in the Now

THERE IS A STORY about a wise indigenous chief who was blind. They say he had the wisdom of Solomon. One day, two young braves came up with a plan to trick the chief and show that he was not so wise or intelligent.

They decided to go before the chief with one of them holding a sparrow in his hand and ask the chief if the sparrow was dead or alive. If the chief said the sparrow was dead, the brave would open his hand and let the bird fly away. If the chief said the sparrow was alive, the brave would crush the bird in his hand; the sparrow would be dead. Either way, the chief would be wrong.

With that plan, the braves went before the chief with one of them holding the sparrow.

"Chief," he said, "I have a sparrow in my hand. Is it dead or alive?"

The chief responded, "The sparrow is as you choose it to be, as you wish it to be."

THE CHOICES YOU MAKE dictate how successful you may be in your caregiving. Many times, you can influence the outcome by controlling the moment, by living in the moment of a person with dementia.

Experts say that exercise is one way to hold off the Alzheimer's monster banging its way out of your closet.[1] It makes sense—do something that raises your heart rate and more blood flows to your brain. In fact, Elaine's doctor says walking is the best exercise for the brain of both a person with Alzheimer's and his or her caregiver. With that advice in mind, one day we set out for a walk on the paved bicycle path behind our condo. Elaine didn't have an agenda. There was no pressure to achieve a goal during what ought to have been a perfectly enjoyable event on its own, and we had no awareness of whether we'd been on that bike path for twenty-one or twenty-three or twenty-nine and a half minutes. However, she was well aware of how tall the trees were, how pretty the flowers were, that there was a butterfly, and that leaves were blowing in the breeze. Her interest was to take in nature's wonders and appreciate them zen-like and in the moment.

My goal was to walk from A to B in thirty minutes, to get it done, and go on with my day.

Checking my watch, mentally moving on to whatever was next on my to-do list when we got home—that was my misguided focus. How foolish of me! I missed a moment of joy. We missed out. The sooner you choose to acknowledge the disease, the sooner you begin to identify and enjoy those moments. It is your choice to enjoy the process—of walking or whatever—without focusing on the end result. I definitely could have made better decisions. I'm telling you, don't wait until it's too late.

So, if it's a beautiful day for a walk, do that. But when the walk is happening, it is your choice either to let an arbitrary fitness standard rule the day or, instead, to capture that moment of joy.

I hope you choose to enjoy the moment and snap a mental picture that you can hold.

Remember the cognitive tests that Elaine was given? She started out with a score of twenty-eight out of thirty points on one assessment. But as the score went down, caregiving responsibilities increased, as did the demand for my attentive response. It's like watching the temperature drop—the colder it gets, the more layers of clothing you need. When you are prepared, moments of joy happen more easily. When you are not prepared, brace yourself for moments of frustration.

While no two people with Alzheimer's experience the disease in exactly the same way, it is in the late stages that a person undergoes the greatest changes in physical abilities. Bicycling was a hobby that Elaine and I enjoyed over the years, and that bike path behind our condo is so conveniently located. They say you never forget how to ride a bike, right? Well, they're wrong. Elaine got to the point where she could no longer ride a bike.

So we went to a bicycle shop that sold three-wheel models, designed for adults with balance difficulties. Elaine was successful sitting on the bike, but because her Alzheimer's was so far advanced, she couldn't relate to the handlebars. She could not comprehend that if you wanted to go straight you held the handlebars steady in front of you. "This is stupid," she announced, getting off the bike. I had no idea how dramatically she could decline. By the time I'd thought of the three-wheeler, her tests were scoring in the low teens. The disease was just progressing too quickly.

What I Wish I'd Known

Alzheimer's is a disease of inactivity of both mind and body. As it progresses, the person with the disease becomes slower and less capable. You can try familiar activities, but you need to accept when the brain can no longer process the information.

Trying to get Elaine to ride that bike was a product of my living in the past. It was as illogical as expecting her to be able to handle trips to Boston and Florida. I had lived such an active life with my First Elaine. With my Second Elaine, that is no more. Unfortunately, it took me too long a time to realize that I must choose to let go, to accept that hard truth. We still can experience happiness, but like Dorothy in *The Wizard of Oz*, we must find it right in our own backyards.

One of the most painful losses for couples affected by Alzheimer's is not being able to really talk about the kids and grandkids. Milestones such as graduations, weddings, and births come and go. Sadly, a person with Alzheimer's is unable to be truly involved. For them, those family members might as well be strangers off the street.

Knowing that, I do tell Elaine about our children and grandchildren. It's still worth doing. She might not be able to relate to the characters in my stories all the time, but she can sense that these are people I love and am proud of. She can feel the joy I am expressing. It's not the details of the stories that are important; it's the mood that is created by telling them.

That's my way of slaying the dragon: choosing to see my wife as the person she is now. Helping her enjoy the person she is now. Helping her sense that I am happy to be with her now. I've finally learned to slow down and appreciate the moments of joy, however fleeting they might be. Thankfully, most of the time she still knows me and always remarks about how good-looking and intelligent I am. Who wouldn't want to hear that?

I never want to pass up the opportunity to tell Elaine how pretty she is, how wonderful she is, what a good person she is. She likes that. Sometimes when I do that, she calls me a BSer again, but we both laugh and enjoy the moment. Her smile tells me she is in a good place.

The person my wife is now finds happiness in lots of things. We listen to music and sing. We play catch. We play board games without rules. We color—we were way ahead of that coloring-books-for-adults fad! And we make simple art projects. (An Alzheimer's Association program called Memories in the Making helps persons with the disease express themselves through art. The watercolor paintings they create are remarkable and so good they can sell at auction for several hundred dollars.)

What I Wish I'd Done

By wishing for the past, I had deprived my wife of happiness in the moment. Even though it broke my heart, I should have let go of my First Elaine sooner so I could love my Second Elaine where she is now.

I know Elaine benefits from the comfort and security that come from just being with me and other people who love her, including the people she gave her life to. Everyone deserves that bit of dignity, regardless of his or her mental condition. I still need her, and she somehow knows that. She's sensitive and aware of her surroundings. After sixty-one years of marriage, she's closely tuned in to my attitude, frustration, and impatience; she seems to know precisely what emotional state I am in.

We spend a lot of time just looking out the window. It's an experience much like that walk on the bike path.

"Look at that tree. It's so big!"

"The sky is so blue."

"Those are pretty flowers."

And then we start over with our little survey of nature until she finally loses interest. You have to grasp each of those statements and appreciate them individually, not dread the tedium of it. What she had for dinner isn't on her mind right now—her mind is focused on the thought that the tree is big, the sky is blue, the flowers are pretty.

Go to your kitchen or your workbench, get a funnel, and hold the narrow opening up to your eye. When you look through the narrow end of the funnel, that's the world as you usually see it—going from a small tunnel to a widescreen view. Your world is full of motion, and interesting. Now, turn the funnel around and look through the wide mouth. The perspective is flipped. That's the way someone with Alzheimer's views the world. It starts out big, then narrows to that small opening. The peripheral things drop away, and those with Alzheimer's see—with laser focus—only what's right in front of them. Learning about Alzheimer's, choosing to enter the world of a person with dementia, and adapting how you interact with your partner are wise steps for you to take. They give comfort to your partner, are necessary parts of coping, and help you survive as a caregiver. It is as your partner would choose it to be, as he or she would wish it to be. It is as you should choose it to be, as you should wish it to be.

PART 3

Surviving
Alzheimer's Disease

Life is good and I plan to have it continue that way until my children tell me it's time for a nursing home or something like that. This is realistic with what my Alzheimer's book says about my future. But 'til then, I will try my best to be normal—whatever that means—and keep my happy side of life always continuing. I'm lucky to have such a good family and many friends to help get me through all this. And so, another great day to thank the Lord and smile, smile, smile.

—ELAINE'S NOTES DURING A VISIT TO
DOOR COUNTY, WISCONSIN, JULY 3, 2012

CHAPTER 10

———⊗⊗⊗———

Challenges

AS A YOUNG STATE senator, I regularly heard one of the leg-islature's most bombastic orators. He was a legend in his own mind. He came from the western part of Wisconsin, along the Mississippi River. He bragged in his speeches about the "courage, fortitude, and conviction" of his constituents when dealing with the spring floodwaters of the mighty Mississippi.

Well, this silver-tongued senator passes away, and he's met at the pearly gates by Saint Peter. "New arrivals have to give a speech," Saint Peter says. The senator, with great confidence, tells Saint Peter he will once again deliver his speech about the courage, fortitude, and conviction of his constituents as to how they dealt with a flood along the Mississippi River in the spring-time.

"That's well and good," says Saint Peter, "but I want to warn you: Noah and his three sons will be in the audience."

WHO AM I TO be talking about pain and hardship when you may be going through something much worse?

As challenges go, I'd like to think I've done all right. I accept

the fact that I'm a work in progress. Not even Noah got everything right—he brought geese onboard, and we all know what a
mess they can cause.

As I've climbed this mountain, I've succeeded in tiptoeing
around some of the goose piles created by Alzheimer's and
stepped smack-dab into others. Maybe you can learn from my
mistakes. My hope is that our discussion here can help you survive and be the best possible caregiver for your own situation.

What I Wish I'd Known
When your partner gets an Alzheimer's diagnosis,
it's important to get started on a bucket list of things
you want to experience together. Prioritizing helps
you feel comfortable later on when you are alone and
must do things without your spouse.

Elaine and I are eighteen years into this so-called journey.
Some of the worst days are behind us.

I've received the phone call from my bewildered wife, lost
while driving, surrounded by orange construction barrels, and
trying to explain herself to a police officer. I've answered the
same questions for her every five minutes. I've seen her confuse
lipstick with nail polish and helped her when she couldn't figure
out how to put on her bra. I've given away most of her clothes
and her car.

None of that was pleasant.

But in so many ways, as the psalmist wrote, "My cup runneth
over" (Psalm 23:5).

We have terrific kids who love their parents very much. Even
though our daughters live more than a thousand miles away,

they visit often. All the kids come at the drop of a hat if I ask them or need them. Our grandchildren and great-grandchildren impress me with their talents and passions and inspire me to work toward a world without Alzheimer's for their generations.

We're blessed to live in a major urban area with access to great medical care and other resources that make a world of difference in Elaine's well-being and mine. I'm lucky enough to own a business. I can set my own hours and work from home. I can delegate responsibilities to a team I have trusted for years. When I require time off to devote to Elaine's needs, my business partners understand and cover for me so I don't have to worry about the day-to-day routine. Actually, the firm has done better without me and grown. I thank them for their great support and friendship.

If any of our employees are ever put into a caregiving situation—Alzheimer's-related or not—I'll have insights into the added challenges they are facing. I want to be understanding of their divided attention and give them the opportunity to carry out their responsibilities without worrying that their career will suffer.

I can only hope you are managing things. Nationwide, more than one-third of Alzheimer's caregivers reduce their hours at work or quit their jobs to provide care, losing an average of $15,000 in annual income.[1] How can they possibly absorb a financial hit like that? The Alzheimer's Association's 2016 Special Report provided some bleak answers: to make ends meet, one in five caregivers cuts back on his or her own doctor visits, and 11 percent don't get all of their own medications. The situation can be so dire that these heroes are 28 percent more likely to eat less or go hungry.[2]

The report also talked about "care contributors," defined as people who frequently or occasionally pay dementia-related expenses, provide care, or do both. These generous friends and family members spend an out-of-pocket average of more than

$5,000 annually for groceries, medical supplies such as adult diapers, and in-home care. The price tag is many thousands more if the person with dementia lives in a care facility—maybe as much as $100,000 a year.[3] Many people assume that Medicare, Medicaid, or basic health insurance will cover nursing home costs, and sadly, that's not the case. No wonder that 70 percent of people with Alzheimer's are cared for at home.[4]

I know I am so, so fortunate in that I had purchased long-term care insurance for both of us, which allowed Elaine to receive excellent day-care services for nearly four years, and now allows her to be cared for in an outstanding assisted-living facility. Only 7.2 million American adults have such insurance.[5] I'd like to think that being in that slim minority means I'm smart; in fact, this is the result of a principled, persistent, pestering, almost obnoxiously unbearable life-insurance agent. (You know who you are, and I luv ya, kid!) That decision, years ago, has assured that Alzheimer's care won't bankrupt us.

So don't feel sorry for me.

My heart aches for you because you're just getting started. Your life's circumstances may be a lot more difficult than mine. Maybe you were struggling even before your spouse was diagnosed. Maybe your loved one has younger-onset Alzheimer's (also known as early onset), adding to the shock and sadness of your situation. Maybe you have health problems of your own. Maybe you don't have a good relationship with your children (or don't have children at all), so you lack that younger, more energetic supportive presence in your life. Maybe you live in a smaller community where the nearest adult day-services program is an hour away. Maybe there are financial difficulties. Maybe it's some other misery or daily strain.

Any one of these challenges is reason to reach out—and I mean now—for help in surviving.

What I Wish I'd Done

I should have forgiven myself for not being perfect. I was doing the best I could in a difficult situation. It's understandable to have regrets about my shortcomings, but there is no point in feeling guilty.

If you ever hear of someone who is completely successful, healthy, and happy as an Alzheimer's caregiver by going it alone, let me know. That person should be written up in the medical journals and maybe even considered for sainthood.

I never realized how bad I had gotten until I overheard a phone conversation with whomever you were talking with on the phone, and I'm sorry to make life so difficult for us, and I guess I don't fully understand how difficult I've been for you. . . . I don't want to be a burden to you anymore. You deserve much more, and I understand. And I want to thank you for all you have done for me and love you forever.

—A NOTE FROM ELAINE TO MARTY,
DATE UNKNOWN

CHAPTER 11

What Surviving Looks Like

Y EARS AGO, I WAS flying early one morning on a business
trip from Milwaukee to Washington, DC, and as I got on the
plane, a well-dressed, distinguished gentleman was speaking to
the flight attendant. He was explaining to her that he needed her
help because he had to get off the plane during its stopover in
Detroit, and he was worried he might sleep through it. "Of
course," the flight attendant said, "I'll make sure to wake you. I
promise. I guarantee it." To my surprise, as everyone got off the
plane in Washington, who should I see but that well-dressed
gentleman. His behavior was anything but distinguished—he
was yelling and complaining at the flight attendant as he stormed
away. I couldn't help but feel sorry for her. "My goodness," I said,
"that man was so angry."

She replied, "He's angry? You should have seen the fellow I
put off the plane in Detroit."

LIKE THAT DISGRUNTLED PASSENGER, when Alzheimer's en-
tered your life, you were taken to a destination you did not
choose. I didn't pick it either, but now that I have journeyed

up that rocky mountain, I know where—and why—I made mistakes.

By now, I hope I've succeeded in telling you that to be a successful, loving caregiver, you need to first *learn* about the disease. Doing so makes it possible to *cope* with the heroics of caregiving. The third part of my mantra is *survive*.

I can be considered a survivor of Alzheimer's because it is a disease with two patients: the person with the diagnosis and the caregiver. I also use the word *survivor* because I anticipate I'll outlive Elaine. In a way, I already have. I am a widower with a wife.

As a survivor, I'm more sensitive to, and understanding of, what it means to lose someone you love. I'm more aware of other people's feelings, their challenges, their pain.

Survival is about peace of heart, knowing I've done all I could, including writing this book to hopefully help other caregivers. It also means I'm taking the time—and now I have the time—to be a better parent, a better grandparent, a better friend, and a better helper to others in this life. Once you've dealt with and adapted to the challenges of this dreaded disease, every role you play becomes more meaningful.

I survived the early stages of this disease when Elaine's behavior first pointed to trouble. I survived the transition from spouse to the ever-changing role of caregiver. I survived the heartache of watching the disease progress. Surprisingly, no one actually did punch me in the nose due to my irrational irritability.

In the middle stages of the disease, as I mentioned earlier, Elaine's sleep patterns made it impossible for me to get a decent night's rest. Sometimes, she'd be out of bed and wandering around the condo. She wasn't sure which door was to the bathroom and which one led outside. There's a busy street a block from our driveway, and Lake Michigan is just two blocks away. Knowing she could get lost in our home, I feared what she would do if she got outside. I had an extra lock put on the door, and I started sleeping on the couch. I hoped that if Elaine did try to leave, I would hear her and could protect her from any harm.

At my age, night after night of poor sleep—in fact, year after year—took an insidious toll. My exhaustion and frustration became so severe that I had little left to give when the disease progressed to the late stages.

One day about eight years after Elaine's diagnosis, I was finishing a phone call with our daughter Kathy. "I love you," I said as I told her goodbye. Elaine overheard this and wanted to know who was I talking with, and I told her it was our daughter Kathy. "We don't have a daughter named Kathy," she insisted. "Why would you make that up?" Her tone was most uncharacteristic, hostile and accusing. She insinuated that this Kathy had to be someone who was not to be associated with. "You've got to be up to no good," she said. She wanted to know who else I was in love with. I knew it was the disease talking and not Elaine. She was the one who had told me that you can lose an election but you can't be defeated. This outburst, however, did defeat me. I began to seriously wonder, *How much longer can I live with my wife, and how much longer can she live with me?*

After loving Elaine for sixty-two years, I was angry with myself for even thinking this way.

I LOVED SAILING FROM a young age. When we were in high school, I bought a rowboat, wanting to make it my very first sailboat. Elaine went to the Army surplus store and bought old parachute fabric that she fashioned into sails. As often happens, one boat led to another. Eventually, we owned real sailboats, one of which we named *True Love*, inspired by an old movie called *High Society*. In it, Bing Crosby sings a love song to Grace Kelly:

Suntanned, windblown
Honeymooners at last alone
Feeling far above par
Oh, how lucky we are

While I give to you and you give to me
True love, true love
So on and on, it will always be
True love, true love

Six months a year, we'd be out on the waters off Milwaukee and, farther north in Wisconsin, off the Door Peninsula. On a sailboat, you're in the elements, which is fun when you're young and romantic, and you go where the wind takes you. What great times! As the years went by, we traded the labor of sailing a boat for a forty-six-foot cruising trawler that we named *Beyond Ayes* because it represented a life beyond anything I thought I would ever have.

We had the adventure of a lifetime on that trawler, with our friends Judy and Ron—a five-thousand-mile trip we did in segments from 2005 through 2007. On a route called "America's Great Loop," we rode the current through Illinois and south on the Ohio River and the Tennessee–Tombigbee Waterway to Mobile, Alabama. From there, it was around Florida, and then we motored up the Eastern Seaboard at seven knots to the Hudson River, the Erie Canal, the Great Lakes, and home again. We shared the Mississippi River with barges full of coal and passed by the Statue of Liberty. We celebrated the success of my cancer treatments, and we ate well and laughed so much. But even then, uncertainty was creeping in when Elaine did some strange things, like putting the salt and pepper shakers "away" in the oven. Little did we realize that the odd behaviors were early symptoms of Alzheimer's.

Our boat has been our second home. Over Memorial Day weekend in 2015, the four of us went out on the water together for what proved to be the last time.

I was hoping the long holiday weekend on the boat would be just as enjoyable as the Great Loop trip a decade earlier. I could catch up with Judy and Ron, and they could help keep an eye on Elaine. But even in that small space, Elaine got lost. In the middle of the night, Ron woke me to say Elaine had come to their tiny sleeping quarters, asking, "Where is Marty?" She'd had to climb over me to leave our bed! I'll never know what possessed her to do that, and I shudder to think what would have happened had she gone out onto the deck. That told me just how rapidly the disease was progressing. I could never leave her alone. Never. It was time for Elaine to live elsewhere. Yet I still felt guilt.

What I Wish I'd Done
I wish I would not have let my ego get in the way of what was best for Elaine.

My counselor at the Alzheimer's Association had opened the conversation a year earlier. "When the time comes," she said, "you are not 'putting' her in a nursing home. You are not 'putting' her anyplace. Her illness is causing her to have more needs than one person can handle, even with adult day care and in-home help. You cannot respond to all of her needs. A dementia care unit can, with trained staff who are new and fresh every eight hours. You will be giving her an opportunity to be at the best place she could be."

She wasn't the only one suggesting a move for Elaine. Many others had been asking why Elaine was still living at home. That's the toughest question a caregiver has to face—ironically, sometimes it comes from the very people who doubted the Alzheimer's diagnosis in the first place. But you know me: I'm stubborn.

Moving to a facility was never going to cure Elaine. I knew that. But I also recognized that Marty's One-Man Nursing Home was no longer good enough either. That realization made it somewhat easier for me to accept the inevitable: Elaine should move. After all, to quote a seventeenth-century poem I read in high school, "stone walls do not a prison make."[1]

Our children and I did some research, taking tours of care facilities and asking a lot of questions. We watched to see how attentive the staff was and whether the residents seemed interested in the activities that were offered. We were lucky to have options, including the two facilities where Elaine had most recently attended day programs. After weighing the pros and cons of the facilities, we arranged for Elaine to move to the residential memory unit of the same place where she first attended a day program.

None of that made it any easier when The Day came.

It was horrible to take her there. I remember so well the day after Labor Day in 2015. As we left our home, she accidentally left the door open as she followed me out into the attached garage. I didn't have the heart to tell her to close the door behind her because it marked the end of that life as we knew it. Instead of taking her to the adult day-care center where she'd gone five days a week for the previous two years, we drove ten miles to her new home. It is a caring, compassionate place. She deserves nothing less. Her room is comfortable but small, with the intent that she spend most of her day with other residents and in activities. In advance, we had hung family photos in hopes of giving her touchstones to her past.

The facility's staff advised me to avoid visiting for the first five days so that Elaine could become acclimated. It was difficult to be separated from her, but I had to trust that it was best for her. We did talk on the phone a couple times. They showed her a short video I had recorded in which I told her I was busy in Madison and would see her soon. A bit of therapeutic fibbing.

Even as I adjusted to the emptiness in my home and in my heart, there were two emotions dominating my thinking: relief that Elaine would be safe and hope that now I could focus on being a better father and grandfather. It was like competing in a relay race. You run your hardest, and then you hand off the baton to someone with strong, untired legs. Let's face it—you're never going to find someone who says, "Hooray for me! I put my wife in a nursing home!" But I do know this: we both are in a better place. I now get a better night's sleep. I get my exercise. I have a better chance of being healthy. And I no longer worry every minute about Elaine.

I visit her almost every day, and I am learning to not feel guilty when I don't. She deserves my best attention, and she picks up on it if I'm preoccupied. When I'm overstressed, I'm better off—and more importantly, she's better off—if I stay away.

What I Wish I'd Known
Visiting Elaine when I'm feeling stressed doesn't do either of us any good.

As a person with late-stage Alzheimer's, there is a silver lining in this very dark cloud that envelops Elaine. It's that she lacks awareness of all she's lost: her independence, her memories, her future. She is not upset by the fact that she lives in a care facility and wears an adult diaper. And because she is no longer anxious, neither am I.

The less she knows me, the less she demands of me. It is my hope that she is experiencing a familiar voice, one that makes her feel comforted. I make a point to tell her what a wonderful wife, mother, and grandmother she is. I thank her for all she's done for me.

Now Elaine has advanced to the severe stages of Alzheimer's. But up until then, we still enjoyed car rides and dining out. We were limited only by my imagination and energy. When we walked around the shopping mall near her care facility, we saw lots of young children. In those moments, she'd hand out compliments as readily as she did at the Wisconsin Executive Residence or in her preschool classroom. "You're a cutie," she'd say. That was my Elaine.

Even after Elaine went into assisted living, I still felt her presence so strongly in our bedroom that for almost a year I continued to sleep on the couch. I eventually decided to make a clean break from some of the bad memories by moving into a smaller, ground-floor condo in our complex. A home without stairs is a good thing for someone who's had all the health problems I've had.

Home, I've learned, isn't a building. It's a place inside you where you feel secure. That goes for both of us.

Elaine now lives across town from me. She has left our condo behind for good. She lives just a couple of miles from Milwaukee Lutheran High School, where we spent our first years together. In a way, we've come full circle.

I am so very lucky I met Miss Elaine Ruth Thaney in freshman Latin class, lucky to have her fall in love with me, lucky she said yes, lucky she supported every dream and crazy idea I ever had, lucky she raised such great kids, lucky I still get to hold her hand every day. If Alzheimer's is the worst thing that can happen to me, I've got the best of the worst. For what better blessing, better promise, can any person receive . . .

When in heaven, I will always be smiling down at you.

With great love to the best man in the world.

—ELAINE'S NOTE TO MARTY, 2015

If Alzheimer's Could Speak

Talk to me...
  I can hear your words and they still touch my soul.

Smile at me...
  My eyes can see you and feel your heart even if I don't remember how to smile back.

Hold my hand...
  I can feel your energy when our hands connect. It makes me feel safe and less alone.

Love me...
  My heart can feel your love even if my words can't express mine.

Live your life...
  Help me on my path but don't press pause on your life. Be the vibrant person I know & love.

Trust the process...
  I know this is hard and not what we planned but trust the process. We can't control it but we can choose our focus. Remember the good times, know that I am ok and that you are in my heart always.

—TARA REED

Afterword

S UCCESS IN THE CASE of Alzheimer's caregiving is a nebulous and relative term. Anyone who has lived through it knows Alzheimer's disease takes an enormous toll on people with the disease and is devastating to caregivers on many levels—emotionally, physically, and financially. However, in the course of my work as the executive director of an Alzheimer's Association chapter, I saw that those best able to move forward in the caregiver process were able to accomplish something that I began to think of and call "the pivot."

In regard to the partner who has dementia, the pivot is about reaching a point where the caregiver is able to emotionally let go of the person he or she knew before and move into a new relationship with the person the loved one is becoming as the disease progresses. Literally pivoting away from the old and toward the new.

This pivoting is one of the hardest human undertakings I have witnessed. The person you pivot away from may have been your husband or wife, the mother or father of your children, your soulmate, the person you rely on to share burdens and make your way through life. Perhaps cruelest of all, the person who played those roles in your life is still physically there before you but unable to continue behaving in the same ways.

In the face of this dynamic, most caregivers spend years trying to make the person with the diagnosis "try harder" or "concentrate more," which makes both people feel awful and changes nothing. Those who accomplish the pivot (and it's not a one-time thing—it's more like a skill that becomes more familiar the more it's practiced) are able to enter into a new way of relating to their loved one, and even a new era in the rest of their lives.

No one that I know of has done a better job illustrating how the pivot works than Marty Schreiber in this book. At its core, his is a love story that continues to this day. And the very title speaks to the all-important necessity of letting go to be able to move ahead.

I think it's important to note that gaining the wisdom Marty shared here almost cost him his life. The stresses of caring for Elaine and emotionally adjusting to her Alzheimer's landed him in the hospital more than once. But he came out of the experience with a passion to do all he could to help other caregivers—as he puts it, to learn, cope, and survive. I hope that through this book, you've been inspired to follow his navigational light into a new tomorrow.

–Tom Hlavacek, former executive director,
Alzheimer's Association of Wisconsin

Acknowledgments

THE AUTHORS ARE GRATEFUL to their families for their support, encouragement, and invaluable contributions during this project. Marty particularly thanks his children, Kathy, Marty, Kristine, and Matt, as well as Bob and Rose Schreiber, Jill Schreiber, and Bill and Marion Schreiber. Cathy thanks her husband, Kent Lowry, and daughter, Greta.

Marty also thanks his business partners at Schreiber GR Group (formerly Martin Schreiber & Associates, Inc.) for their extraordinary patience and friendship and gives special thanks to Denise Cifaldi for helping in countless ways. We know that writing this book took longer than we told you it would, so thanks for hanging in there.

Thank you also to Tom Hlavacek, Lynda A. Markut, Mary Ann (Miller Vance) Clairday, and the entire staff of the Alzheimer's Association Southeastern Wisconsin Chapter. They cheered us on every step of the way.

Many others helped by editing the manuscript without destroying our spirits, including Judy Banta, Betsy Benson, Bill Christofferson, David Cross, Hugh and Mary Denison, Jim Haney, Al and Anne Iding, Tom Krajewski, Lynn Krebs, Fred and Coleen Latzke, Kelsey Lawler, Ron and Judy Lokken, Anita and Bob Pietrykowski, Kate Huston Raab, Sue Schalk, Bob Schulze, Pete Schumacher, Don and Karen Six, Ann Stacy, Edie Starrett, Tom and Sue Thaney, John Vitek, Ralph Weber, and Maria Welk.

I want to acknowledge the team at Elaine's Hope Memory Care and Assisted Living Facility with admiration and gratitude for their compassion, patience, and loving care of Elaine. In particular: Ruthie Adams, Carey Bartlett, Kathy Cavers, Trinie Davies, Mark DeGuzman, Kaila Kaddatz, Stephanie Leanes, Jackie Marks, Scott McFadden, Mary Orr, Linda Oster, Rachel Payne, Alicia Prince, Danielle Rombca, Julie Shanley, Ingrid Stoffel, Lourdes Suarez, Tysheena Sykes, Senait Teklezghi, Dyonne Wilhelm, and Derek Wolter, chaplain.

We also honor the memory of Kitty Rhoades, former secretary of the Wisconsin Department of Health Services. Kitty was committed to ensuring all whom she served had a voice, especially those suffering from dementia, mental illness, and disabilities.

In addition, Marty thanks caregivers he has met and the authors of the many Alzheimer's-related books. Your insights are making a big difference in people's lives.

Cathy honors family members who have suffered from dementia, including Anna McClintock, Ralph Breitenbucher, Karl McClintock, and Helen Farrar. The loving example provided by their caregivers through the past forty years has been an inspiration.

Resources

Alzheimer's Association
National 24-7 Helpline: 1-800-272-3900
https://www.alz.org

You also can follow the association on Facebook and YouTube (@actionalz), Twitter and Instagram (@alzassociation), and LinkedIn.

Other resources may be available in your area, sponsored by the county, state, or federal government. Services they provide may include:

- information about options for long-term care
- elder abuse and crisis intervention
- information about public and private benefits
- community-based services
- home-delivered meals
- caregiver respite
- transportation

Look for organizations with names such as:

- Aging and Disability Resource Center
- Aging Resource Center
- Area Agency on Aging
- County Department on Aging

You can research nursing homes in your area at https://www .medicare. gov/care-compare. Facilities are given one to five stars as an overall rating, as well as for health inspections, staffing levels, and how well the facility cares for its residents' needs.

Information about adult day care can be found at https://www .communityresourcefinder.org under Community Services. You also can learn more through the National Adult Day Services Association (https://www.nadsa.org).

———∞∞∞———

Q&A Conversations
from the Road

SINCE *My Two Elaines* WAS first published in 2016, I've visited with thousands of Alzheimer's caregivers across the country. I have heard from many caregivers who give of themselves and demonstrate their love and commitment in ways that are almost unbelievable. Nevertheless, some of these heroes tell me they experience overwhelming guilt, resentment, and frustration, and they often feel forsaken by friends. To help offer you sound advice and answers to common questions, I turned to my counselor at the Alzheimer's Association, Lynda A. Markut.[1] Our combined responses are as follows:

Q: *How do I get family members and friends to help more or even just spend more time with our loved one who has dementia?*

A: Lynda provided me her wisdom in a gentle way, but I will be more direct: I have no right to demand that others handle the disease in a manner I dictate. Everyone deals with this loss in their own way. I need to forget about imposing my standard of grieving and coping on others. Ask yourself, *How much time and energy do I have to devote to others' reactions?* Know when to let it go.

Think about what might be at the root of this situation. Children, siblings, or friends may still hold on to the former reality. They want to remember the person with dementia as he or she was, not see the individual as he or she is today. They may even feel they can't deal with visiting someone who has dementia. So teach them more about Alzheimer's. For questions you cannot answer, refer them to the Alzheimer's Association (https://www.alz.org). Even if you continue to disagree about help, visits, and such, do what you can to maintain good relationships with family and friends. Perhaps one silver lining to Alzheimer's is that you may develop valuable new friendships when you participate in support groups and caregiver activities.

Q: *How do I know it's time for my loved one to move to a care facility?*

A: Think of a balance scale. On one side are the needs of the person with dementia—on the other are the needs of the caregiver. What is the benefit to your loved one of living at home versus the physical and emotional strain imposed on the main caregiver? Is the person with dementia negatively impacted by the caregiver's stress and poor health? Does he or she require care you simply cannot provide at home? Pay attention to how much the scale tips. Working with an Alzheimer's counselor or listening to experienced caregivers in a support group can help you work through your emotions.

Transitions are difficult for both a person with dementia and his or her caregivers. No one wants to leave his or her home. Take some small steps to help your loved one adjust to spending time away from you. Care at home, day care, and twenty-four-hour in-home care can be successful options long before the need for a nursing home. When you research various types of care, you make better decisions. A loved one who feels you are trying to convince him or her will push back. Say something like, "We're going to try this. The doctor says it's a good idea." Always put things in a positive light.

Q: *Why do I feel so guilty?*

A: Guilt comes from the absolutes we put in our heads, such as promising you will never put someone in a nursing home. Situations change, so "never" no longer applies. Let go of any guilt weighing you down. Even though you sometimes become frustrated, angry, and impatient, realize that such feelings are normal. You have done and are doing your best to make your loved one as comfortable as possible.

Q: *How have your kids handled all this?*

A: For years I was so focused on my struggles that I simply didn't ask them, and I regret that. Now I'm getting a better understanding of what our children have been dealing with. Here are some of their thoughts:

> KATHRYN LYON: At first, I was burdened with self-doubt about our phone calls, obsessing about how often and when I called, what questions I asked Mom, what information I gave her. After each call, I would judge the conversation. Did we make a connection? Did we build a new memory or secure an old one? How long did we talk? Did she know she was my mom and I was her daughter? Over time, I realized I could not hold on to my mother as I remembered her. I no longer try to remind my mother that I am her daughter. Now our conversations are about the two of us meeting in the moment as friends and sharing who we are right then and there.

MARTIN R. SCHREIBER JR.: I was both relieved and sad when we decided to move Mom to memory care. I know it was very difficult for Dad. I'm sure, in a certain sense, it was like saying goodbye to their life together. Today, in the advanced stages of Alzheimer's, Mom provides a perfect example of what I should do when I am with her—simply smile and share each present moment. She may not know who I am, but she can certainly feel love and kindness.

KRISTINE HAAS: Realizing my mom had Alzheimer's was a brutal reality on many fronts. First, the grief of losing my mother—albeit piece by piece—was real, slow, and painful. Second, watching my dad try to figure out how to manage this new situation was tricky. Many times, I knew my dad needed help, but I didn't know how to give it. It also took Dad a while to be able to accept the help he needed. Third, living with the understanding that my chances of getting the disease are higher makes me look at life differently. I often need to remind myself to push away the fear and replace it with hope while living each day to the fullest.

MATT SCHREIBER: When I learned my mom had been diagnosed with Alzheimer's, it wasn't a surprise. I had seen her memory slipping slowly for years. However, I was ignorant about what Alzheimer's really was. What worried me was not only how it affected Mom but also how it was taking its toll on my father and in turn the family. Now when I visit her, I don't have any expectations of her knowing who I am. You can see that she values the company, which is more important to me than her knowing who people are.

Q: *Doesn't it hurt you when Elaine no longer recognizes you?*

A: Yes, it was extremely painful. It would have been so much better for me had I understood and accepted earlier that there were two Elaines. Now, in the late stages of the disease, the Second Elaine tells me, "I love you more than my husband." That tells me our souls are connecting.

On our wedding anniversary, I spent extra time with Elaine. After having dinner together, I helped her into bed and sat next to her, holding her hand and thinking of our life together. I began to cry, and Elaine asked me what was wrong. I told her, "I just want you to know I love you very much."

"Okay," she said. "Then everything is good."

Q&A Between Marty
and Dr. Michelle Braun

DR. MICHELLE BRAUN IS a board-certified neuropsychologist who is passionate about empowering individuals to boost brain health and reduce the risk of Alzheimer's with science-backed strategies.[1] Her work has been featured on PBS, NPR, CBS, FOX, iHeartRadio, and in other media outlets. She completed her internship at Yale School of Medicine and postdoctoral fellowship at Harvard Medical School/Boston VA. She previously served as the assistant director of inpatient mental health at the Boston VA and instructor of psychiatry at Harvard Medical School. Dr. Braun has a popular blog on brain health in *Psychology Today* and has been a member of the Scientific and Advisory Panel of the Wisconsin Alzheimer's Association since 2005. Her bestselling book, *High-Octane Brain: 5 Science-Based Steps to Sharpen Your Memory and Reduce Your Risk of Alzheimer's*, empowers readers to optimize brain health and well-being with an inspiring personalized action plan and tracking system.

MARTY: For our friends who may not be familiar with your wonderfully helpful book, *High-Octane Brain*, can you tell us a bit about your work?

DR. BRAUN: I so appreciate you asking about *High-Octane Brain*, as in many ways it's the embodiment of my passion over the past sixteen years. After I started my clinical practice in 2005, I noticed that my patients were unknowingly using unproven strategies to improve their memory, including supplements, online brain games, and restrictive "brain health" diets.

In addition to using unproven strategies, I noticed that many patients were relying on strategies that are minimally helpful, such as crosswords or sudoku puzzles. It was heartbreaking to see many people—including those with a family history of Alzheimer's—investing time and money into strategies that weren't truly effective.

It was even more heartbreaking to know that many people in the community and worldwide didn't have direct access to a professional they could ask about brain health strategies. This disconnect between the desire to improve brain health and the knowledge of proven techniques ignited my passion to share scientifically based information more widely. I started a *Psychology Today* blog on brain health in 2017 and began the process of interviewing top researchers to write *High-Octane Brain*.

The book includes interviews with eight top brain health researchers and nine brain health role models ages 44 to 103 and combines their insights with the latest science into a personalized tracking system to enhance brain health and reduce the risk of Alzheimer's. It's been exciting to share this information with the public. What I especially love is that the same strategies that maximize brain health often maximize happiness. It's a win-win!

MARTY: "Brain health"—that seems to be something many take for granted until it's too late. Tell me about your experience with brain health. I understand that you're a neuropsychologist. I know that's not a medical doctor, so what is a neuropsychologist?

DR. BRAUN: A neuropsychologist (not to be confused with a neurologist or with a psychologist, who focuses on psychotherapy) is a medical provider with a doctoral degree who specializes in the diagnosis and treatment of disorders that impact brain functioning—including Alzheimer's and other types of dementia.

As we know, the brain controls not only our thinking skills (otherwise known as our cognitive functioning) but also our emotions, motor skills, social skills, and ability to perform daily tasks. Neuropsychologists specialize in using statistically based tests that measure the "software" of the brain: skills such as memory, attention, multitasking, language, decision-making, visual ability, motor functioning, judgment, and emotional functioning. Interestingly, even though many of these tests might appear to be "lower tech" (because they are done verbally and on paper), they are as accurate as blood tests and brain scans!

Neuropsychologists combine cognitive test data with the results of medical tests (like brain scans and blood tests), medical history, observations during the examination, and reports from the patient and caregiver to provide an accurate diagnosis. That diagnosis then serves as the basis for a personalized treatment plan that includes not only medical management strategies but also recommendations to minimize future cognitive decline, maximize daily functioning, and enhance quality of life for the patient and caregiver. It additionally provides a valuable baseline for tracking future cognitive and behavioral changes.

The goal is to provide an integrated, holistic, science-backed plan of action. What I particularly love is that every plan is tailored to the patient, their caregivers, and family. In a sense, the plan aims to help the patient and family understand what they can be at their best and connects them with needed resources to achieve their highest possible level of cognitive, emotional, and daily functioning.

MARTY: In my experience as a caregiver, this holistic approach you describe is incredibly essential—and it really does involve not only the person with Alzheimer's but also the caregiver, family, friends, community, and resources at large. What would you say are the most important things a caregiver should know from the start when learning of their loved one's diagnosis?

DR. BRAUN: I think it's important for caregivers to know that the experience is akin to embarking on a journey that will change who they are, in ways that may be challenging and painful and also in ways that can be surprisingly positive.

Caregivers often find it helpful to know that others have traveled this journey before and that they can benefit from those insights. As with any journey, learning as much about it as possible ahead of time is helpful. That's where health-care professionals, support groups, resources like the Alzheimer's Association, and books like *My Two Elaines* can be immensely helpful.

I encourage caregivers to envision their health-care providers as part of the team that will travel their journey with them. I also like to offer to initiate contact with the Alzheimer's Association on behalf of a caregiver through the Direct Connect program, so that they feel supported throughout their journey.

MARTY: Well, you're certainly the gold standard of medical professionals then, Dr. Braun. In my experience and in what I hear from other caregivers, medical professionals can, at times, be tricky to deal with—whether it's lacking bedside manner, not giving enough information, or relaying unhelpful information. When a caregiver accompanies their loved one to the doctor, what are the key questions they should ask?

DR. BRAUN: I think working with a medical professional that specializes in Alzheimer's is vital—so for starters, determine whether your loved one is working with an expert. You can certainly ask the medical provider about this directly, but you might even consider first connecting with the Alzheimer's Association or a support group to solicit feedback about recommended experts in your region.

One of the advantages to working with an expert is that there is often less pressure on you to ask the "right" questions. An expert will proactively provide you with information and support. However, it can always be helpful to ask for any clarification you might need regarding issues related to diagnosis and recommended treatment.

For example, inquiring about whether treatment options include medication and behavioral strategies can be helpful, as the most effective treatments often involve both components. Exercise, social engagement, and cognitive engagement, as well as some types of medication, have been shown to slow the rate of Alzheimer's for some individuals.

It's also important to clarify whether you can call your health-care provider to address concerns or distressing issues that might arise between appointments.

Finally, ask how you as a caregiver can best help the health-care team. What kind of information would they find most helpful from you? If you find yourself in the unfortunate situation where you feel there is not a good fit with your loved one's health-care provider, don't hesitate to discuss your concerns with the provider directly or ask others for recommendations. Trust and partnership with your loved one's health-care provider are essential to maximizing their experience and your caregiving journey.

MARTY: So just as support from the health-care provider is essential, I find that support from family and friends is equally crucial to success as a caregiver. Many people claim they have no idea how challenging it is to be a caregiver. What do you believe is the most important way in which family, friends, and neighbors can lend support and give emotional strength to the caregivers in their lives?

DR. BRAUN: I do think it's impossible to know what it's truly like to be a caregiver unless one is a caregiver. Friends and family must start by acknowledging that. They might also ask how the caregiver feels about the caregiving role itself and validate those emotions. A caregiver might feel intense sorrow about the changes their loved one is exhibiting and how that is impacting their relationship. They might feel envious of others who do not have to be caregivers or guilty that they resent aspects of the caregiving role. They might feel anxious and ill-equipped to be a caregiver. They might feel deeply lonely, as if no one could possibly understand what they are going through. And the truth is, no one but the caregiver truly does understand what they are going through. It can be a powerful act of caring for the caregiver to validate their emotions and emphasize that they are normal reactions to being thrust into one of the toughest roles imaginable.

Perhaps the caregiver would like you to attend a support group with them or a seminar at the Alzheimer's Association to learn more about the condition and how you can stay involved and supportive. Perhaps they would benefit from having you spend time with their loved one while they take a much-needed break. Acknowledging the work that a caregiver is doing, initiating frequent check-ins, and offering to help in tailored ways that address their needs are all great ways to provide support. Listening is key.

Sometimes we see that caregivers establish new friendships in support groups with other caregivers who more innately understand their experience, so keeping an eye out for new opportunities to develop friendships can also lead to increased support.

MARTY: To dig a little deeper into this dynamic between caregivers and their social circle, we've established how common it is for friends and family to remove themselves from the world of the person with Alzheimer's. For instance, when the person with Alzheimer's has moved to assisted living memory care, longtime friends, brothers and sisters, even their own children don't come to visit.

Some rationalize this choice, saying, "The person with Alzheimer's wouldn't recognize me anyway." But this lack of support and showing up affects the caregiver just as much, if not more, than the person who has the diagnosis. Do you have any advice for caregivers who feel forsaken? How might we shift our thought processes to cope with the absence of family and friends? How might we approach them about their choice to stay away?

DR. BRAUN: I'm so glad you asked this question because, as you mentioned, this experience is unfortunately very common for caregivers, and it often intensifies caregiver distress and loneliness. In caregiver support groups, we frequently discuss the loneliness and disconnection that caregivers experience when family, friends, and other loved ones decrease or even discontinue contact or when they misunderstand or misattribute the symptoms of a loved one with Alzheimer's or other dementia.

What I've noticed is that long-standing personality traits often impact the way that family, friends, or other loved ones engage in support and caregiving. Just as our family and friends have varying levels of insight regarding their own personality traits and a varying sense of empowerment regarding their ability to change their own behavior, they also often have variable insight regarding the need to be present as a caregiver and a variable sense of empowerment about their ability to provide support and care.

Researchers often refer to an individual's sense of empowerment to change events in their lives as "locus of control." Individuals with an internal locus of control feel empowered to change their future experiences through internal efforts, such as their own actions or willpower, whereas individuals with an external locus of control feel that external forces, such as luck or situational factors, determine their fate.

Individuals with an internal locus of control are often more naturally engaged in the caregiving experience, perhaps because they feel that what they do will make a difference to them and their loved one. In addition to locus of control, personal tolerance of distress may impact caregiving engagement. For example, there may be a preference to remember the person "as they were" prior to experiencing symptoms of Alzheimer's or other dementia rather than witnessing changes that could be distressing .

One way to address the impact of disengaged loved ones is to share how you feel and let loved ones know you miss their presence. I've noticed that disengaged loved ones are often surprised to learn that there is a desire for them to be more present and supportive.

It can also be helpful to provide disengaged loved ones with tailored, concrete suggestions about how to provide support—whether that is having a loved one attend a support group with you, read a book (like *My Two Elaines*) to obtain education and caregiving ideas, provide meals, or visit more frequently. In addition, initiating a discussion to understand why a disengaged loved one has been less present may help to highlight underlying assumptions and quell fears (e.g., "I don't want to get in the way" or "I wouldn't know what to say").

But keep in mind that, ultimately, the way a disengaged loved one responds to a request to increase support or caregiving engagement often varies due to personal factors that are long-standing and not specific to the caregiving experience.

MARTY: It has been my experience that caregivers become so strongly focused on and engrossed in caring for their loved one that they often exclude almost everything else in their lives—like going to the gym, meeting with friends, taking a break. It seems like caregivers need to get permission from someone to even laugh. Any advice to caregivers who seek permission and affirmation?

DR. BRAUN: Yes, it's typical for caregivers to prioritize caregiving to the extent that they minimize or discontinue their own self-care. It's often a gradual process that seems to increase over time—a missed break here and there that becomes the norm.

My advice is to prioritize at least thirty minutes of time per day for self-care from the outset of the caregiving journey. This may sound like a lot of time, but discussing with your support team how they might help you prioritize this can make all the difference. Maximizing your "well-being buffer" with exercise, social activity, and engagement in activities you enjoy is not only therapeutic for you but is also a means to enhance the quality of your interactions with your loved one.

MARTY: I know I've learned that it's not only the waking hours that support self-care but the sleeping hours too! I'm reminded of a line in Max Ehrmann's 1927 poem "Desiderata," which goes: "Many fears are born of fatigue and loneliness." What tips can you share for caregivers who don't get enough sleep?[2]

DR. BRAUN: What wise words! I think sleep, like food, is key to building our "buffer" in daily life. Our reactions to situations are markedly different when we have rested, had a sandwich, and taken a step back to think through a situation versus when we are not well-rested, hungry, and stressed.

As you mention, good sleep can be particularly difficult for caregivers. A helpful first step can be to figure out the cause of poor sleep and to enlist a health-care provider in that discussion. Perhaps there is an undiagnosed sleep disorder that could be treated, or a medical condition that is causing poor sleep that could be treated (for example, many people with chronic pain don't sleep particularly well).

It can also be helpful to schedule a "wind-down" routine prior to bedtime. Think of the hour before sleep as an opportunity to train your brain to prepare for sleep: shut off blue-light devices (like televisions, smartphones, and computers) and do something relaxing (such as reading, praying or meditating, or taking a warm bath). If you aren't able to fall asleep after ten minutes (which is common for caregivers, who may be thinking about all they need to do next!), it can be paradoxically helpful to get out of bed and do something relaxing—such as reading or listening to music—and then return to bed when you feel fatigued.

By doing this repeatedly as needed, you can retrain your brain to associate lying in bed with sleeping rather than thinking. Increasing your activity level during the day (for example, exercising regularly) can also enhance sleep. In turn, better sleep sets in motion a positive feedback loop by decreasing the likelihood of depression and improving mood.

MARTY: Speaking of depression and mood—in my mind, I'm convinced that caregivers experience an unacknowledged grieving. It's unacknowledged by family and friends, even unacknowledged by caregivers themselves. This, I think, subconsciously weighs very heavily on the mind of the caregiver, who sees their loved one die a little bit every day but with no acknowledgment of the loss. Talk to me about this. Is there a way of helping caregivers deal with this? Am I right in my assumptions ?

DR. BRAUN: Yes, it's very common for caregivers to experience grief. It may not be noticeable on a daily basis, but it often grows over time and in retrospect may be clearer.

Unacknowledged grieving is so common that it has been studied by researchers and is referred to as "ambiguous grief." Ambiguous grief refers to the gradual losses that can occur in the context of dementia, including changes in the relationships, roles, personality, and activities that were once characteristic of a person. Perhaps a loved one who used to cook, sing, or hug no longer engages in those activities, which were core to their identity.

That shift is often accompanied by the sadness and grief of caregivers and loved ones, though the grief is ambiguous because the loved one is still alive and the closure that is typically associated with grief is not possible. Because caregiving can sometimes feel like a journey of successive losses, it's important to be aware of and validate ambiguous grief and to give yourself space and time to discuss and process your emotions.

MARTY: I imagine that from this ambiguous grief also comes an unacknowledged depression in caregivers. I certainly can see why a caregiver would become depressed, due to the worry of what the future might be while also realizing and experiencing a daily loss. What can we do about that?

DR. BRAUN: One way to decrease the likelihood of depression is to address it proactively and discuss the possibility of it before it occurs. This is one reason that support groups, loved ones, and health-care providers on your support team can be especially helpful to you from the outset. Your support team can help decrease the frequency and severity of any depression you might experience by staying in contact, initiating discussion, and helping you process disappointments and challenges before they become significant.

Proactive self-care—including exercising, participating in enjoyable events, getting adequate sleep, and processing your emotions with trusted others—also helps to decrease depression.

MARTY: Perhaps to help caregivers deal with these feelings of grief and depression, we could talk about one of the core emotions that leads to the rest of them. In my experience, caregivers often feel a burdening sense of guilt, even as they do their heroic work. Why do you think that is?

DR. BRAUN: I've noticed that as well. I wonder whether there is an inherent tension between the devotion that caregivers have to ease the suffering their loved one is experiencing and the reality that even the best caregiving techniques are imperfect at alleviating suffering. So on one hand there is a powerful drive to help in the best way possible, and on the other hand there is a daily witnessing of challenge and, often, decline. This inherent dilemma may inadvertently lead caregivers to blame themselves.

In other situations, caregivers tell me they feel guilty that they don't understand what their loved one needs, or they feel mixed emotions about their loved one as the relationship shifts. Sometimes there is also a desire to take a break from caregiving, which can fuel a sense of guilt. Over the years, I've heard many reasons why caregivers feel guilty, and the reasons are as complex and individual as caregivers themselves.

Connecting with other caregivers to discuss guilt and other challenging emotions can be incredibly validating and healing. That's one of the many reasons I love your book so much. By sharing your insights and experiences as a caregiver, you open a space for reflection, discussion, validation, and ultimately, acceptance of the inherent dilemmas present throughout the caregiving journey. You also give voice to the realization that love—and decisions based on that love—is the most valuable caregiving intervention.

MARTY: Thank you for your kind words—getting to this point has certainly been a journey. When it comes to making decisions out of love, there's one that, to me, stands above the rest. It's one of the toughest things a caregiver has to do—and it's also one of the things which will most help both the caregiver and the person who is ill to live their best lives possible.

The caregiver must let go of the person who once was, to embrace and care for the person who now is. I've experienced this firsthand. My friend Tom Hlavacek, the former head of the

Alzheimer's Association of Wisconsin, calls it "the pivot." What kind of advice can you give to help caregivers conquer that extremely difficult act of deciding to let go?

DR. BRAUN: "The pivot" is exceptionally difficult. As you mentioned, it requires letting go of who a person once was and embracing who they are in the moment and who they will become. I believe the caregiving journey requires a succession of thousands of tiny pivots over time. It can be helpful at the beginning of the caregiving journey to discuss and normalize the process of pivoting so that caregivers are alert to small changes. Doing so provides an opportunity to identify not only the challenges inherent in pivoting but also the periodic positive aspects of pivoting.

For example, many caregivers tell me that they've been surprised to see their loved one experience a sense of peace due to "living in the moment" more frequently than they previously had (of course, this is not always the case).

And pivoting often occurs for caregivers as well. For example, some caregivers, in reflecting on their journey, have shared that they feel more direct in their communications with other people and more focused on maximizing their experiences because they have a deeper appreciation of the value of time.

MARTY: I can relate to that. But also, as I've shared with my friends, I've sent too many boxes of candy and bouquets of flowers as a result of what I have come to term "irrational irritability." Help me with this.

DR. BRAUN: I believe "irrational irritability" is a rational and normal reaction to the disappointment and loss that caregivers feel at many points of the caregiving journey. Irritability, irrationality, anger, grave disappointment, intense sadness, and a host of other unpleasant emotions are common and even expected when witnessing a loved one decline or encounter significant challenges.

Recognizing those emotions is key. This is where a support team of other caregivers and health-care providers is crucial. I can't tell you how many times I've heard caregivers sigh with relief when they hear other caregivers discuss a similar perspective, a shared experience, or how they, too, have dealt with unpleasant emotions. There is often great solace in knowing that we are not alone in our pain and disappointment. Your story provides that validation for so many.

MARTY: It's reaffirming to hear that, so thank you, Dr. Braun. In that vein, I'd like to dive a little deeper into my story, if you don't mind, and speak with you about some moments I've experienced firsthand while caring for Elaine. In sharing these experiences, my hope is that my fellow caregivers can feel even more that they are not alone in the challenges they face every day.

For instance, in my book I talk about a time when I realized I should have employed "therapeutic fibbing." Elaine had asked me how her parents were and became shocked and anxious when I reminded her that her parents were both dead. When would you say is the right time for a caregiver to transition from reality into therapeutic fibbing?

DR. BRAUN: This is such an important question because situations often arise when a loved one asks about a topic they have forgotten about but are likely to be distressed by. Individuals with dementia are especially likely to ask about their parents or siblings, given that childhood memories are strongly etched in the brain. It can be similarly challenging to know whether to mention recent events that could be troubling to your loved one, such as an upcoming funeral, a pandemic, or an illness that the caregiver is experiencing.

"Therapeutic fibbing" involves communicating in a way that prioritizes your loved one's peace of mind, and as such often involves not mentioning information that is likely to be distressing. The intent is not to lie or mislead for self-serving reasons but rather to share information in a way that your loved one can process with minimal distress, especially given that the ability to process distressing emotions is often impaired in dementia. Individuals with dementia are also often impaired in their ability to reflect and think critically about the context of a distressing event. To use your example, all they are hearing in the moment is, "Your mother passed away."

In contrast, although people who do not have dementia may feel extremely sad when remembering the death of a loved one or reflecting on a negative event, they are often able to think through the information in a way that considers multiple facts and eventually alleviates their distress—for example, they may recall that their loved one was relieved of the pain they were experiencing before they died or that their loved one lived a long and fulfilling life. But imagine how traumatic and shocking it would be if you were told that someone you believe to be alive actually died years ago, and you did not have the cognitive ability to put that information into context. Tragically, that's often how people with dementia experience distressing information.

The timeline for using a "therapeutic fib," as well as the content of the "therapeutic fib," will often depend on your loved one's ability to process information. It can be helpful to ask clarifying questions (e.g., if your loved one asks, "Where is my mother?" you might respond by asking, "Where do you think she might be?"). The answer can help you to shape your ultimate response.

MARTY: That is such wonderful and practical advice. But it can be particularly difficult when it's not just a difficult question being asked but a distressing claim or accusation, such as "you are unfaithful" or "you never come to visit" or "you stole my money." How would you recommend a caregiver respond to a distressing claim that isn't true?

DR. BRAUN: Rather than disputing the content of a distressing claim or accusation (which can be frustrating for caregivers and for the individual with Alzheimer's or other dementia), it is often best to help the individual focus on something different. This can sometimes be done by changing the topic of discussion.

Other techniques include engaging in a sensory activity that your loved one enjoys, such as listening to music, looking at a photo album, eating a snack, swaying/dancing to a favorite song, rubbing your loved one's back, or brushing his or her hair. Enjoyable sensory activities often stimulate the emotional center of the brain (limbic system) and as such provide a strong emotional stimulus that can sometimes override the emotion of the accusation.

If there seems to be a common time of day or situation in which the accusations occur (e.g., in the afternoon, directly after a visit has started or is about to end), it can be helpful to proactively engage in an enjoyable activity to see if that might minimize the accusations. If changing the subject or engaging in a sensory activity doesn't appear to be helpful, consider changing the physical environment, perhaps by relocating to a nearby room, going outside, or taking a walk. Sometimes a change of scenery can do wonders for prompting a shift to a more positive topic.

Keep in mind that if none of these strategies seem to work, it can be helpful to retry the same strategy—or a new strategy—on another day. Trust your instincts, and experiment with different strategies (and/or different timing of similar strategies) to see if they might work.

MARTY: On the flip side, what if the inaccuracy isn't so big and distressing but rather small and mundane? How much correcting should a caregiver do? For example, when being called by the wrong name or when the discussion doesn't fit reality as far as time, place, or activity. My personal opinion is that it depends on where my loved one is mentally and emotionally on any given day. But usually, I find a caregiver should "roll with it." Isn't that the best thing we can do for a person with Alzheimer's? To join their world, wherever their world may be?

DR. BRAUN: I agree! Joining the world of your loved one and "rolling with it" is a perfect way to honor their emotions and perceptions as they may change on any given day and keeps interactions from becoming habitual. In general, I recommend that corrections be minimized unless there is a safety issue involved, given that the act of correcting information can draw attention to an error and unwittingly may lead a loved one to experience shame and guilt for misremembering. This might also lead a loved one to converse less due to fear of misremembering and reduce overall dialogue, which is the opposite of what we are trying to encourage. Furthermore, corrective information is not likely to be remembered.

One strategy I've found helpful when responding to misremembered information is to ask an opinion-related question. For example, if your loved one references a dinner the night before and says, "I loved the dinner we had last week," rather than gently correcting the statement ("Oh yes, I loved the dinner too, but it was actually last night, not last week"), it may be helpful to ask, "What did you like about the dinner?" This type of open-ended, opinion-related question minimizes a focus on facts, keeps the conversation flowing, and allows us to learn more about our loved ones.

MARTY: That flow of conversation reminds me of a time when Elaine and I were having lunch, and she started to cry. When I asked her what was wrong, she said she was beginning to love me more than her husband. Well, I did not ask her, "What's wrong with your turkey husband?" But it certainly had an impact on me. My takeaway was that it was not necessary for her to know who I am in order for our hearts to touch. Can you tell me what might have been going on in Elaine's mind? What is the most comforting thing I could have said or done? And what comfort can you give to a caregiver whose lifetime together with a loved one seems to be being erased?

DR. BRAUN: That's so powerful. It sounds like Elaine was speaking to you from her heart and voicing your deep emotional connection, which transcended her factual understanding of who you were to her in that moment. As Alzheimer's progresses, it can impact the ability not just to recognize and remember the names of familiar faces but also to remember aspects of one's personal identity, life experiences, and relationships. I'm wondering if Elaine cried because she was attempting to reconcile the love she was feeling toward you with her belief in that moment that you were not her husband and perhaps feelings of sadness because she was also aware of the deep love that she feels for her husband.

Thankfully, a recent study in which individuals with dementia provided feedback about what they found to be emotionally meaningful can give us some guidance about how to navigate such situations. Individuals with dementia reported that they felt more connected and valued when a caregiver attempted to share moments of emotional connection with them, and when caregivers supported their ability to communicate by connecting with them physically, emotionally, and verbally, and empathizing with what they were feeling in the moment. Powerfully, even when caregivers were unable to fully understand what a loved one was trying to communicate, their attempts to connect emotionally were felt and valued by loved ones with dementia.[3]

You are so adept at connecting with Elaine that I have a feeling you responded in a way that gave her great comfort. I think connecting with her through touch (perhaps holding her hand) and talking with her about the love she was feeling—without correcting her perception of who she thought you were in that moment (unless it was distressing to her not to have you do so)—may have given her comfort in the midst of her sadness. She may also have been touched to learn about your love for her.

Promoting and treasuring moments of emotional connection—even if they may be infrequent and include different types of connection than have historically been shared—can help to offset the feeling that one's life experiences with a loved one are being erased by the disease.

MARTY: It's true. I've seen firsthand just how important that emotional connection is. Though I admit, at times, I am plagued by Elaine asking the same question over and over and over and over and—well, you have the idea—again. How should a caregiver handle repeated questions? I tell you, it can be exasperating.

DR. BRAUN: Yes, even though we intellectually understand that repeated questions are a common symptom of dementia, it can be exasperating to experience them. A few things can be helpful. First, investigating the reason behind the question can be useful. For example, your loved one may be asking a question not because they actually want it to be answered but perhaps because they want to engage socially or minimize boredom. One way to test this is to see whether engaging in an activity, touching your loved one, or listening to music or watching a movie minimizes the questions.

If it appears that your loved one is asking a repetitive question for the purpose of having it answered, it can be helpful to write the answer on a small portable whiteboard or notebook (which your loved one can be encouraged to take wherever he or she goes). Then, you can cue your loved one to look at the written information anytime the question is repeated. Because motor memory skills (e.g., looking at a whiteboard or notebook) are generally easier to remember than factual information, after this is practiced several times, your loved one may eventually start to look at the written information without you needing to prompt and without repeating the question aloud to you. Another bonus of this technique is that your loved one might experience improved mood due to greater self-reliance and might start writing important information down.

MARTY: Along the same lines, how should one handle their loved one's involuntary, repeated calls for "Help, help" or "I want to go home!" At times it seems no soothing a caregiver can think of will stop these pleas, unfounded though they might be.

DR. BRAUN: I'm so glad you asked this, because repeated calls for help can be quite distressing for caregivers to witness, especially when no amount of soothing seems to minimize them. First, it can be helpful to explore the meaning behind this behavior with the same spirit of curious inquiry that you use to investigate the meaning behind a repeated question.

For example, repeated calls for help may signal an unmet need that cannot otherwise be communicated. Perhaps your loved one is in pain; is bored, hungry, or thirsty; needs to use the bathroom; wants to interact; or is experiencing physical discomfort due to the temperature in the room or uncomfortable clothing. Because there are so many potential underlying reasons for repeated calls for help, it can be useful to determine if there is a pattern to the behavior that can clue you in to the underlying need.

The ABC (Antecedents, Behavior, Consequences) model, developed by Dr. Albert Ellis, is a great method to help address such behavioral challenges.[4] You can begin the process by writing down the "Antecedents" to your loved one's concerning behavior (i.e., whatever is happening before the behavior begins). For example, you might note the time of day, the people in the environment, the time since your loved one last ate or used the bathroom, your loved one's position while sitting or lying down (does he or she look physically comfortable?), or any variety of other factors that you can observe.

Next, write down the details of the concerning "Behavior." For example, what are the exact words your loved one is saying, and is your loved one doing anything when he or she says them? Is your loved one awakening from sleep, shifting his or her body in pain, turning away from a light source, etc.?

Lastly, write down the "Consequences" that result from the behavior. For example, does the behavior result in others interacting by touching, soothing, or providing a drink? Responses that result in attention, interaction, touch, food, drink, or meeting other needs might unwittingly be increasing the repeated calls for help, but they also provide important clues about how to meet the underlying need (which might benefit from being proactively attended to).

Feel free to ask for assistance from friends and professionals when using the ABC model, given that observations from trusted others often provide novel insights into the reasons behind a behavior and may expand on what you notice. Once you better understand what could be giving rise to the concerning behavior, you can put tailored strategies in place to minimize it.

In addition to using the ABC model to develop personalized behavioral management strategies, general soothing strategies may also be helpful. These might include playing your loved one's favorite music, providing a soothing tactile object (e.g., a favorite pillow or blanket), providing something to care for (a doll or a stuffed animal "pet" such as a dog or cat), posting pictures of family members, or "simulated family presence" (playing a tape of you and/or family members conversing, which your loved one can listen to when you are not physically present). A spirit of curiosity, investigation, and creativity is often key to uncovering the underlying reasons for repeated behaviors and finding solutions (often developed through trial and error) to minimize them.

MARTY: As we wind down this interview, I'd love to ask you about something I've heard you say. You say that caregiving is an opportunity to see yourself as a new person and that even something good can come out of this experience. I believe there is life after death—but life after Alzheimer's? That's sort of tough for me to see right now. We caregivers can't imagine that something good can come out of this experience, so where did you get that from?

DR. BRAUN: I'm currently in my fifth year of cofacilitating a dementia caregiver support group, and I've been fascinated to hear the evolving perceptions of caregivers as they reflect on different stages of their journey. Although each caregiver's journey is unique, there seem to be some overlapping commonalities. In the earlier stages of the journey, there is often a focus on the "nuts and bolts" of becoming a caregiver, which may include becoming educated about the disease, connecting with a health-care team, and engaging their loved one in supportive services.

As the journey progresses and caregivers observe sometimes heart-wrenching changes in their loved ones' personalities, it is common to see the "ambiguous grief" that we talked about previously. Simultaneously, some caregivers notice unexpected positive changes in their loved ones, such as a greater focus on the present moment or a decrease in previous anxiety or depression.

Caregivers also frequently report unexpected positive changes in their own personality, which they often attribute to caregiving challenges. For example, they may experience a clearer sense of the fragility of life and the value of time, such that a previous focus on meeting societal expectations is replaced by engaging in more authentic relationships. Many caregivers also report a newfound appreciation of their own resilience and a deeper sense of empowerment. In addition, because many caregivers also become advocates for their loved ones, it is not uncommon to hear them discuss new ways they have learned to advocate for themselves and others.

Even in cases where a loved one passes on, several caregivers have stayed active in our group and express a deep desire to support other caregivers. Although the journey of a caregiver is not one that would be chosen by anyone, and the heartbreak and loss is often devastating, there may still be some deeply positive changes that result from the journey.

MARTY: Thank you for that reminder, Dr. Braun. Well, we've covered a lot of territory. What are your final thoughts as I strive to be an outstanding caregiver? To sum up, my own thoughts would be to join the world of the person who now is. To be courageous and intelligent enough to ask for help. To get enough sleep, exercise, and decent nutrition, and to plant positive thoughts in your mind. Am I on the right track?

DR. BRAUN: I don't think I could say it any better, Marty. Yes, yes, and yes to all of the wisdom and insights you've shared! Joining the world of your loved one as the moments unfold second by second, with a focus on the present moment, is so powerful and so respectful of your love. It also allows infinite opportunities to tailor communication and activities to what your loved one is experiencing and keeps the interactions fresh.

There is also much to be said for engaging in joint activities that provide you and your loved one with enjoyment, such as listening to music, looking at pictures, reading together, doing puzzles or crafts, and spending time with family. As you mentioned, self-care is essential to well-being, and is also foundational to the ability to provide your loved one with the best care. In addition to good sleep, healthy food, and exercise, spending regular time in calming environments—for example in nature, church, or a library—can be rejuvenating.

One thing that can also be very therapeutic and enhance a sense of purpose and happiness for your loved one is to see how they might respond if you give them something to care for, whether that is a pet, a plant, a doll, or even a robotic animal (interestingly, robotic animals are often popular among individuals with dementia). Providing multisensory engagement can also enhance well-being. For example, exploring your loved one's preferences as they relate to smell (e.g., pleasant-smelling foods and candles), touch (e.g., soft, comfortable textures), sounds (e.g., music or calming background noise), sight (e.g., calming pictures and views of nature), and movement (e.g., swaying, dancing, or walking) can also enhance happiness and quality of life, especially as memory and language skills shift over time.

Thank you, Marty, for your devotion to sharing your insights and easing the journey for countless caregivers. Your love for Elaine shines through in all you do and inspires us all!

Notes

FOREWORD

1. Alzheimer's Association, "2021 Alzheimer's Disease Facts and Figures," *Alzheimer's & Dementia* 17, no. 3 (March 2021): https://doi.org/10.1002/alz.12328.

INTRODUCTION

1. *Morning Edition*, "Forget Lincoln Logs: A Tower of Books to Honor Abe," NPR, February 20, 2012, https://www.npr.org/2012/02/20/147062501/forget-lincoln-logs-a -tower-of-books-to-honor-abe.
2. Alzheimer's Association, "2021 Alzheimer's Disease Facts and Figures."
3. Alzheimer's Association.

CHAPTER 2: DIAGNOSIS

1. Alzheimer's Association, "2021 Alzheimer's Disease Facts and Figures," *Alzheimer's & Dementia* 17, no. 3 (March 2021): https://doi.org/10.1002/alz.12328.
2. Alzheimer's Association, *2015 Alzheimer's Disease Facts and Figures* (Chicago, IL), https://www.alz.org/media/documents/2015factsandfigures.pdf.
3. Vanessa Caceres, "What Does Your MMSE Score Mean?," Caring.com, accessed September 28, 2021, https://www.caring.com/examinations/what-does-your-mmse -score-mean.
4. "Medical Tests for Diagnosing Alzheimer's," Alzheimer's Association, accessed September 28, 2021, https://www.alz.org/alzheimers-dementia/diagnosis/medical _tests.
5. Tanner Jensen, "Origins of Alzheimer's: The Life and Research of Dr. Alois Alzheimer," Being Patient, August 29, 2019, https://www.beingpatient.com/alois -alzheimer-life-and-research/.

6. "Key Statistics for Childhood Cancers," American Cancer Society, last updated January 12, 2021, https://www.cancer.org/cancer/cancer-in-children/key-statistics .html.

7. National Institute on Aging and the World Health Organization, *Global Health and Aging* (Bethesda, MD: National Institutes of Health, October 2011), 6, https://www .who.int/ageing/publications/global_health.pdf.

8. "Life Expectancy," Centers for Disease Control and Prevention, April 9, 2021, https://www.cdc.gov/nchs/fastats/life-expectancy.htm.

9. America Counts Staff, "2020 Census Will Help Policymakers Prepare for the Incoming Wave of Aging Boomers," United States Census Bureau, December 10, 2019, https://www.census.gov/library/stories/2019/12/by-2030-all-baby-boomers -will-be-age-65-or-older.html.

10. "Development & Approval Process, Drugs," US Food and Drug Administration, January 7, 2019, https://www.fda.gov/drugs/development-approval-process-drugs/.

11. "NIH Clinical Research Trials and You: The Basics," National Institutes of Health, October 20, 2017, https://www.nih.gov/health-information/nih-clinical-research -trials-you/basics.

12. Jeffrey L. Cummings, Travis Morstorf, and Kate Zhong, "Alzheimer's Disease Drug-Development Pipeline: Few Candidates, Frequent Failures," *Alzheimer's Research & Therapy* 6, no. 4 (July 2014), https://doi.org/10.1186/alzrt269.

13. Christopher Melinosky, "Which Medicines Treat Dementia?," WebMD, August 9, 2020, https://www.webmd.com/alzheimers/guide/medicines-to-treat-dementia

14. Cummings, Morstorf, and Zhong, "Alzheimer's Disease Drug-Development Pipeline."

15. Robert Mitchell, "The Democrat Who Cried (Maybe) in New Hampshire and Lost the Presidential Nomination," *Washington Post*, February 9, 2020, https://www .washingtonpost.com/history/2020/02/09/new-hampshire-ed-muskie-tears-primary/.

CHAPTER 3: DANGER ON THE TRAIL

1. Alzheimer's Association, *2019 Alzheimer's Disease Facts and Figures* (Chicago, IL), 33, https://www.alz.org/media/documents/alzheimers-facts-and-figures-2019-r.pdf.

2. "How Many People Work at Walmart?," Ask Walmart, Walmart (website), accessed September 28, 2021, https://corporate.walmart.com/askwalmart/how-many-people -work-at-walmart.

3. Alzheimer's Association, *2019 Alzheimer's Disease Facts and Figures*, 33.

4. Alzheimer's Association, 70.

5. Alzheimer's Association, 31.

6. Alzheimer's Association, 31.

7. Gail Hunt, Carol Levine, and Linda Naiditch, *Young Caregivers in the U.S.* (Bethesda, MD: National Alliance for Caregiving, September 2005), 5, https://www.caregiving .org/wp-content/uploads/2020/05/youngcaregivers.pdf.

8. "Home Health Aide Training Requirements by State," PHI, 2016, https:// phinational.org/advocacy/home-health-aide-training-requirements-state-2016/.

9. Alzheimer's Association, "2021 Alzheimer's Disease Facts and Figures."

10. Carol J. Farran and Eleanora Keane-Hagerty, "Twelve Steps for Caregivers," *American Journal of Alzheimer's Care and Related Disorders & Research* 4, no. 6 (November 1989): https://doi.org/10.1177/153331758900400608.

11. "Chronic Stress Puts Your Health at Risk," Mayo Clinic, July 8, 2021, https://www.mayoclinic.org/healthy-lifestyle/stress-management/in-depth/stress/art-20046037.

12. Earle Holland, "Chronic Stress Can Steal Years from Caregivers' Lifetimes," Ohio State News, September 17, 2007, https://news.osu.edu/chronic-stress-can-steal-years-from-caregivers-lifetimes---091807/.

13. Alzheimer's Association, *2019 Alzheimer's Disease Facts and Figures*, 38.

CHAPTER 4: ISOLATION

1. Leland Kim, "Loneliness Linked to Serious Health Problems and Death Among Elderly," University of California San Francisco, June 18, 2012, https://www.ucsf.edu/news/2012/06/98644/loneliness-linked-serious-health-problems-and-death-among-elderly.

2. Dan Russell, Letitia Anne Peplau, and Mary Lund Ferguson, "Developing a Measure of Loneliness," *Journal of Personality Assessment* 42, no. 3 (1978): https://doi.org/10.1207/s15327752jpa4203_11.

3. Louise C. Hawkley and John T. Cacioppo, "Loneliness Matters: A Theoretical and Empirical Review of Consequences and Mechanisms," *Annals of Behavioral Medicine* 40, no. 2 (July 2010): 218–27, https://doi.org/10.1007/s12160-010-9210-8.

4. Raheel Mushtaq et al., "Relationship Between Loneliness, Psychiatric Disorders and Physical Health? A Review on the Psychological Aspects," *Journal of Clinical & Diagnostic Research* 8, no. 9 (September 2014): https://doi.org/10.7860/JCDR/2014/10077.4828.

5. Julianne Holt-Lunstad et al., "Loneliness and Social Isolation as Risk Factors for Mortality: A Meta-Analytic Review," *Perspectives on Psychological Science* 10, no. 2 (March 2015): https://doi.org/10.1177/1745691614568352.

6. Rose A. Beeson, "Loneliness and Depression in Spousal Caregivers of Those with Alzheimer's Disease Versus Non-Caregiving Spouses," *Archives of Psychiatric Nursing* 17, no. 3 (June 2003): https://doi.org/10.1016/S0883-9417(03)00057-8.

CHAPTER 5: IRRATIONAL IRRITABILITY

1. "Perpetrators of Elder Abuse Are Usually Family Members," National Care Planning Council, August 18, 2016, https://www.longtermcarelink.net/article-2016-8-18-Perpetrators-of-Elder-Abuse-Are-Usually-Family-Members.htm.

2. "Elder Abuse," World Health Organization, June 15, 2021, https://www.who.int/news-room/fact-sheets/detail/elder-abuse.

3. Aileen Wiglesworth et al., "Screening for Abuse and Neglect of People with Dementia," *Journal of the American Geriatrics Society* 58, no. 3 (March 2010), https://doi.org/10.1111/j.1532-5415.2010.02737.x.

4. Center of Excellence on Elder Abuse and Neglect, *How at Risk for Abuse Are People with Dementia?* (Orange, California: University of California, Irvine School of

Medicine, n.d.), http://www.centeronelderabuse.org/docs/PwDementia_Factsheet
.pdf.

CHAPTER 8: THERAPEUTIC FIBBING

1. Naomi Eisenberger, "The Neural Bases of Social Pain: Evidence for Shared
   Representations with Physical Pain," *Psychosomatic Medicine* 74, no. 2 (February
   2012): https://doi.org/10.1097/PSY.0b013e3182464dd1.
2. Diane Ackerman, "The Brain on Love," *New York Times*, March 24, 2012, https://
   opinionator.blogs.nytimes.com/2012/03/24/the-brain-on-love/.

CHAPTER 9: LIVING IN THE NOW

1. Jon Hamilton, "Is Aerobic Exercise the Right Prescription for Staving Off
   Alzheimer's?," *All Things Considered*, NPR, July 18, 2019, https://www.npr
   .org/sections/health-shots/2019/07/18/743189541/is-aerobic-exercise-the-right
   -prescription-for-staving-off-alzheimers.

CHAPTER 10: CHALLENGES

1. Alzheimer's Impact Movement, *The Impact of Alzheimer's on Families* (Chicago, IL:
   Alzheimer's Association, March 2021), https://alzimpact.org/media/serve/id
   /5d77f273d5fc1.
2. Alzheimer's Association, *2016 Alzheimer's Disease Facts and Figures* (Chicago, IL),
   61–62, https://capitolhillvillage.org/wp-content/uploads/2018/11/Dementia-2016
   -facts-and-figures.pdf.
3. Alzheimer's Association, 59.
4. "Safe and Happy at Home," John's Hopkins Medicine, accessed December 6, 2021,
   https://www.hopkinsmedicine.org/health/wellness-and-prevention/safe-and
   -happy-at-home#:~:text=Of%20the%205.2%20million%20people,and%20help%20
   them%20live%20longer.
5. Alzheimer's Association, "2021 Alzheimer's Disease Facts and Figures."

CHAPTER 11: WHAT SURVIVING LOOKS LIKE

1. Richard Lovelace, "To Althea, from Prison," 1649, Poetry Foundation, accessed
   January 29, 2022, https://www.poetryfoundation.org/poems/44657/to-althea-from
   -prison.

APPENDIX A: Q&A CONVERSATIONS FROM THE ROAD

1. Lynda A. Markut, MS, LCSW, serves as education and family support coordinator for the Alzheimer's Association, Southeastern Wisconsin Chapter. She also is a caregiver and the coauthor of *Dementia Caregivers Share Their Stories: A Support Group in a Book* (Nashville, TN: Vanderbilt University Press, 2005).

APPENDIX B: Q&A BETWEEN MARTY AND DR. MICHELLE BRAUN

1. "About," Dr. Michelle Braun (website), accessed September 29, 2021, https://drmichellebraun.com/about/.
2. Max Ehrmann, "Desiderata" (1927), All Poetry (website), accessed January 29, 2022, https://allpoetry.com/Desiderata---Words-for-Life.
3. Sarah Alsawy et al., "'It's Nice to Think Somebody's Listening to Me Instead of Saying 'Oh Shut Up.' People with Dementia Reflect on What Makes Communication Good and Meaningful," *Journal of Psychiatric and Mental Health Nursing* 27, no. 2 (April 2020): https://doi.org/10.1111/jpm.12559.
4. Kirsten Nunez, "What Is the ABC Model in Cognitive Behavioral Therapy?," Healthline, April 17, 2020, https://www.healthline.com/health/abc-model.

Index

About the Authors

MARTIN J. SCHREIBER grew up in Milwaukee, Wisconsin. Inspired by his father's example as a member of the Wisconsin State Assembly and the Milwaukee Common Council, Martin ran for public office even before he had completed law school. In 1962, he was elected as the youngest-ever member of the Wisconsin State Senate. He was elected lieutenant governor in 1970 and, in 1977, became the thirty-ninth governor of Wisconsin. He recently retired from his public affairs firm in Milwaukee and now is an advocate for Alzheimer's caregivers. In addition to caring for Elaine, Martin is passionately committed to speaking out to help caregivers and their loved ones live their best lives possible. He and his wife, Elaine, are the parents of four children: Kathryn Lyon, Marty Schreiber, Kristine Haas, and Matt Schreiber. They have thirteen grandchildren and seven great-grandchildren.

CATHY BREITENBUCHER is a Milwaukee-based writer who can trace her interest in medicine to dinner-table conversations with her parents, who worked as a nurse and a laboratory technician. She is a native Iowan and graduate of the University of Iowa. She had a thirteen-year career as a full-time newspaper sportswriter, highlighted by covering the Olympic Games in 1984 and 1988. Since 1992, she has been a freelance writer for publications such as *People* magazine, *USA Today*, the *Washington Post*, and several Milwaukee-area magazines and newspapers. This is her third book. She is married and has one daughter.